D1400267

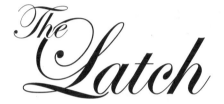

The Latch

and Other Keys to Breastfeeding Success

~

Dedication

For Sebastian and Callista

and

For Adèle, Daniel, Élise and David

~

Acknowledgements

We'd like to thank all the mothers we have worked with who have contributed so much to our understanding of breastfeeding, Diane Wiessinger who wrote so eloquently about breastfeeding as the normal way to feed babies, and Chloe Fisher and Anne Barnes who showed how important an asymmetrical latch is.

Table of Contents

Introduction ix

1. Starting Out Right 1

2. What is a good latch and why is it important? 17

3. Assessing the Latch 47

4. Causes of Latch Problems 61

5. Helping Mothers
   to Learn How to Latch Their Babies 95

6. The Problem of "Not Enough Milk" 103

7. When the Baby Refuses to Latch On 149

8. Healing Sore and Damaged Nipples 159

9. The Premature Baby 165

10. Slow Weight Gain after Initial Adequate Gain 179

11. The Baby Who Refuses to Eat 195

12. Case Studies 203

   Index 217

   Biographies 219

Introduction

Most mothers want to breastfeed their babies. Unfortunately, many of them will end up weaning before their babies are more than a few weeks old. Why? Because they had difficulties – sore nipples, baby not gaining well, baby not latching, etc., etc. – and the health professionals they turned to were not able to help them.

It takes more than a book to reverse that situation. We need health professionals who acknowledge the importance of breastfeeding in infant and maternal health and who will take the time to assess the breastfeeding dyad and teach the mother what she needs to know. We need community and peer support for mothers and families, no matter where they live.

We hope this book will be a beginning, an introduction to some of the keys to breastfeeding success that health professionals need to be aware of as they counsel and support mothers and babies.

The concepts and recommendations here are based on many years of working with breastfeeding mothers and reviewing lactation research. We have seen these techniques work, sometimes dramatically, and we know that with the right kind of help, more mothers can breastfeed longer and more exclusively.

Jack Newman, MD, FRCPC
Teresa Pitman

Starting Out Right

Let me start by saying: there are no benefits to breastfeeding. Breastfeeding is the *natural, physiologic way* of feeding infants and young children, and human milk is the milk made specifically for human infants. There are, however, RISKS to not breastfeeding. Formulas made from cow's milk or soybeans (most formulas, even "designer formulas" and formulas with DHA and other components added) are only superficially similar to human milk, and advertising which states otherwise is misleading.

The slogan "Babies are born to be breastfed" is true in more ways than one. Babies are biologically designed to be ready to feed at the breast and breastfeeding *should* be easy and trouble free for most mothers. A good start helps to ensure breastfeeding is a happy experience for both mother and baby.

Unfortunately, outdated hospital routines based on bottle feeding still predominate in too many health care institutions and make breastfeeding difficult, even impossible, for too many mothers and babies. For breastfeeding to be well and properly established, a good start in the first few days can be crucial. Admittedly, even with a terrible start, many mothers and babies manage to overcome the initial challenges and continue to breastfeed – but others will not be able to or will become discouraged and wean.

The trick to breastfeeding is getting the baby *to latch on well*. A baby who latches on well gets milk without difficulty. A good latch is comfortable for the mother and effective in transferring milk to the baby. A baby who latches on poorly has more difficulty getting milk, *especially* if the supply is low. A poor latch is similar to giving a baby a bottle with a nipple hole that is too small—the bottle is full of milk, but the baby will not get much. When a baby is latching on poorly, he may also cause the mother nipple pain. And if he does not get milk well, he will usually stay on the breast for long periods, thus aggravating the pain. Unfortunately, *anyone* can *say* that the baby is latched on well, even if he isn't. Too many people *who should know better* just don't know what a good latch is.

So how do you get breastfeeding off to a good start? It begins with the birth.

1. Minimize medication during labor and birth. While most pain-relieving medications used during labor are recommended to parents as having no long-term effects on the baby, research shows that, in fact, these medications do affect the baby's ability to coordinate sucking at the breast and, therefore, they may make it harder for the mother to establish breastfeeding. Researchers looking at epidural anesthesia's effect on the baby's breastfeeding skills clearly showed that medication during birth did negatively affect a baby's ability to suckle normally during the first 12 hours and that combining medications increased the effect. Demerol and fentanyl were especially harmful to the baby's suckling ability.

It's clear that, particularly with good help, many mothers and babies are able to overcome this difficult start to breastfeeding. But where other problems are also present, the baby's uncoordinated sucking in the first day or so may be "the final straw."

We also know that when mothers are given intravenous fluids during labor (as they are, for example, when an epidural is given), they may experience edema of the breast tissue (and particularly the areola) which can interact with the fullness caused by the milk increasing in quantity. Usually, the edema begins fairly soon after the baby is born while the increase in milk production happens two or three days after the birth, but they can certainly overlap and cause real difficulties in breastfeeding. Women are often then advised to pump to relieve the pain only to find that pumping simply pulls more fluid into the breasts and makes the situation worse. Avoiding medications such as the epidural which require IV fluids can help reduce this problem as well.

A much more effective treatment for engorgement, especially engorgement that is combined with edema, is Reverse Pressure Softening developed by Jean Cotterman. (See the latest edition of The Ultimate Breastfeeding Book of Answers.*)*

Here's how to do it: Put your thumbs or forefingers, with one on either side of the nipple, near the base of the nipple. Press gently but firmly straight back towards your ribcage. Keep the pressure there for a full 60 seconds. Move your fingers a quarter way around the nipple and apply pressure again.

"Your goal is to create a ring of dimples around the nipple," Cotterman says.

This pushes the excess fluid in the breast tissue temporarily back into the deeper part of the breast so that the baby can more easily latch onto the nipple. It also presses on the milk ducts around the nipple. If they are overly full, some milk may be expressed.

With the breast softer around the nipple, helping the baby latch on well should be easier. Cotterman recommends that mothers use breast compression while the baby is nursing – massaging or pressing on the breast to help the baby get more milk quickly.

If the baby is not able to come to the breast, perhaps because she is ill or premature, Cotterman suggests hand expressing milk rather than pumping.

2. The baby should be at the breast immediately after birth. The vast majority of newborns can be at the breast within minutes of birth. Indeed, research has shown that, given the chance, many babies only minutes old will crawl up to the breast from the mother's abdomen, latch on and start breastfeeding all by themselves. The baby will move to the breast and may start by licking or mouthing the nipple. Usually, he then begins to bob his head as he orients to the nipple and latches on. This process may take up to an hour or longer, but the mother and baby should be given this time together to start learning about each other. The baby can be examined while lying on the mother and other routines can be delayed until after the baby has had time to initiate breastfeeding.

Babies who "self-attach" run into far fewer breastfeeding problems. It also helps the mother feel confident about the breastfeeding process – even if she's not sure how to breastfeed, she can see for herself that her baby is ready and knows what to do.

This process does not take any effort on the mother's part, and the excuse that it cannot be done because the mother is tired after labor is nonsense, pure and simple. All she has to do is lie there and relax while the baby goes to the breast. Incidentally, studies have shown that skin-to-skin contact between mothers and babies keeps the baby as warm as an incubator and reduces any potential drop in blood sugar. Incidentally, it is normal for the blood sugar to drop during the first hour or so after birth so that those postpartum units that do a blood sugar immediately after birth and then an hour or two after and treat a "dropping blood sugar" are treating something that is normal and expected.

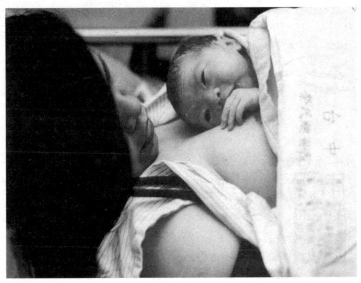

A just born baby skin-to-skin with his mother. Does this look tiring for the mother and the baby?

Some babies do not latch on and begin breastfeeding during this time. Generally, this is not a problem, and there is no harm in waiting for the baby to start breastfeeding when he or she is ready. Simply keep the mother and baby together and be patient. The skin-to-skin contact is good for the baby and the mother even if the baby does not latch on.

By the way, this applies to babies born by cesarean section as well. With a capable person to assist the mother, the baby can be helped to latch on even as the mother's incision is being closed.

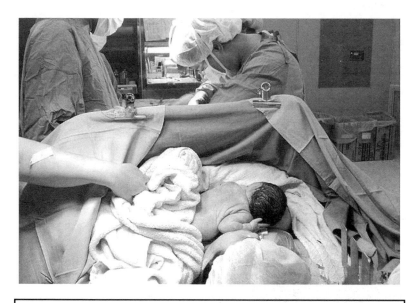

A baby skin-to-skin with the mother while her incision for a cesarean section is being sewn up.

If the baby does not self-attach and/or the mother would like to help the baby latch on, it's essential to be sure that a knowledgeable person is there to provide guidance. Nipple damage can begin with this very first feeding if the baby does not latch on well. The mother may need extra help in finding a comfortable position right after birth, especially if she's had a caesarean section or stitches from a tear or episiotomy. It's important to have someone with the mother who knows how to help a baby breastfeed in a variety of positions.

3. The mother and baby should room in together. There is *absolutely no medical reason* for healthy mothers and babies to be separated from each other, even for short periods.

• Health facilities that have routine separation of mothers and babies after birth are years behind the times, and the reasons for the separation often have to do with letting parents know who is in control (the hospital) and who is not (the parents). Often, bogus reasons are given for separation. One example is that the baby passed meconium before birth. A baby who passes meconium and is fine a few minutes after birth will be fine and does not need to be in an incubator for several hours "observation." Parents make very dedicated observers of their own babies – they will notice every little snort and snuffle. Another common reason for separation is that the mother has a fever and therefore may have an infection which could be passed on to the baby. However, the fever may actually be the result of the epidural she was given in labor – another reason to minimize the use of medication in labor.

• There is no evidence that mothers who are separated from their babies are better rested. On the contrary, they are more rested and less stressed when they are with their babies. Mothers and babies are biologically designed to respond to subtle cues from each other and to sleep in the same rhythm. Thus, when the baby starts waking for a feed, the mother is also starting to wake up naturally. Even when asleep, she is in tune with his quiet noises and is aware of the change in his breathing and the sounds he makes as he gets ready to nurse. This is not as tiring for the mother as being awakened from deep sleep, as she often is if the baby is elsewhere when he wakes up. If the mother is shown how to feed the baby while both are lying down side by side, the mother is better rested.

• The baby shows long before he starts crying that he is ready to feed. His breathing may change, for example, or he may start to stretch. The mother, whose sleep cycles are synchronized with her baby, will be in light sleep, so these small signals will wake her, her milk will start to flow, and the calm baby will be easier to nurse. A baby who has been crying for some time in a room down the hall from his mother before being brought to her and tried on the breast may refuse to take the breast even though he is ravenous. If she does get him on the breast, he may only nurse for a short time before he falls asleep from exhaustion. Mothers and babies should be encouraged to nurse lying down. This is a great way for mothers to rest while the baby nurses. Breastfeeding should be relaxing, *not* tiring.

4. Artificial nipples should not be given to the baby. There seems to be some controversy about whether "nipple confusion" exists. Certainly, it is clear that some babies will show clear preferences for a particular nipple. We all hear about bottle fed babies, for example, who only like one particular brand. Babies are biologically geared to eat, gain weight, and grow. So they will take whatever gives them a rapid flow of fluid and may refuse other nipples that do not.

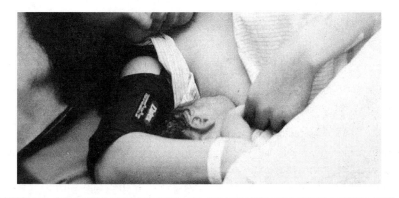

Feeding lying down immediately after birth.

Thus, in the first few days, when the mother is normally producing only a little milk (as nature intended), if the baby is given a bottle (NOT as nature intended) from which he gets a rapid flow of milk, the baby will tend to prefer the rapid flow method. You don't have to be a rocket scientist to figure that one out. Note, *it is not the baby who is confused.* Nipple confusion includes a range of problems, including the baby not taking the breast as well as he could and thus not getting milk well and/or the mother getting sore nipples. Just because a baby will "take both" does not mean that the bottle is not having a negative effect – the baby may not be latching on as well as he could be at the breast. Since there are now alternatives available to bottles if the baby truly needs to be supplemented, why use an artificial nipple?

I think it is important when discussing this with mothers not to call it "nipple preference." Mothers tend to react emotionally to this description, believing that it means the baby prefers the bottle over them. It's more helpful to the mother to explain that we have confused the baby by giving him the fast-flowing bottles, but that her baby really does want to breastfeed.

While pacifiers don't provide milk either rapidly or slowly, there are a number of studies showing that pacifiers reduce the duration of breastfeeding and some suggesting they may also cause latch difficulties. It may be that giving a pacifier means the mother misses some of those early feeding cues described above, so she may feed the baby less often or may end up waiting until the baby is crying with hunger and doesn't feed as well. I've noticed that babies who take pacifiers tend to have more problems with biting down on their mother's nipples as they get older and are teething. They discover that biting on the pacifier is comforting to their sore gums and seem to think they can do the same thing at the breast. (This is not to say that babies who don't get pacifiers never bite – they sometimes do. But the problem seems to be more persistent with babies who get pacifiers.)

5. No restriction on length or frequency of breastfeedings. A baby who drinks well will not be on the breast for hours at a time. Thus, if he is, it is usually because he is not latching on well and not getting the milk that is available. The first step is to fix the latch and use breast compression to get the baby more milk. Compression works very well in the first few days to get the colostrum flowing well. Restricting the length or frequency of feedings will not help this problem. It will also not help the problem of sore nipples, which are most often caused by latch problems.

It is often said that a newborn will nurse an average of 8 to 12 times a day. This does not mean that the baby who nurses 13, 14, 15, or even 30 times a day is in trouble, doing something wrong, or needs to be supplemented as some medical professionals have suggested. We know that in tribal societies, where true unrestricted breastfeeding is practiced, babies nurse an average of 30 or 40 times a day for a few minutes each time, and this may be biologically more normal behavior for infants. As their babies grow, some mothers will want to work towards a more predictable schedule, but at least in the beginning, there should be no restrictions on how often or how long the baby nurses.

6. Supplements of water, sugar water, or formula are rarely needed. Most supplements could be avoided by getting the baby to take the breast properly and thus get the milk that is available. Before considering supplementation, observe at least one feeding at the breast. Work first on improving the baby's latch. This does not mean that the baby should be pulled off and relatched over and over again, as this will just make nipple soreness intolerable for many mothers. Five painful latches cause 5 times as much pain and 5 times as much damage as one. The baby also becomes frustrated as does the mother. A sequence of events occurs that too often results in the baby being fed off the breast, frequently with supplements, to give the "nipples a rest," and too many mothers never overcome this terrible start. The nipples may heal, but often the baby refuses the breast after that. And the latch has not been corrected, so the pain starts again. If the latch hurts, the pain usually diminishes. So leave the mother be, and fix the latch on the other side or the next feeding.

If supplements are required, they should be given by lactation aid *at the breast,* not cup, finger feeding, syringe or bottle. The best supplement is the mother's own colostrum, expressed by hand. (Because the volume of colostrum is small, hand-expression often works best in the first few days.) If there is not much colostrum, it can be mixed with 5% sugar water to be given to the baby. By giving it to the baby at the breast, the baby not only receives the extra fluid but is encouraged and rewarded for nursing at the breast. Formula is hardly ever necessary in the first few days.

7. Be aware that many "contraindications to breastfeeding" are not valid.

Under some circumstances, it may be impossible to start breastfeeding early. However, most "medical reasons" (maternal medication, for example) are *not* true reasons for stopping or delaying breastfeeding. Consult the current issue of *Medications and Mother's Milk* by Dr. Thomas Hale for detailed discussions of the safety of maternal medications – you will find that, in fact, **the vast majority** are safe while breastfeeding and, in many other cases, safe alternatives are available.

Premature babies can start breastfeeding *much, much* earlier than they do in many health facilities. In fact, studies are now quite definite that it is *less stressful* for a premature baby to breastfeed than to bottle feed. Kangaroo Mother Care should be the standard of care for a stable premature baby, and this facilitates breastfeeding as well.

A good start makes breastfeeding easy and comfortable for mother and baby, and it is worth taking the time to help because so many future problems can be prevented.

The importance of skin-to-skin contact

We now have a multitude of studies that show that mothers and babies should be together, skin-to-skin (baby naked, not wrapped in a blanket), the baby's neck extended slightly so his head is in "sniffing position" immediately after birth, and they should spend as much time together skin-to-skin as possible in the days that follow. The baby is happier, the baby's temperature is more stable and more normal, the baby's heart and breathing rates are more stable and more normal, and the baby's blood sugar levels are better. Not only that, skin-to-skin contact immediately after birth allows the baby to be colonized by the same bacteria as the mother. This, plus breastfeeding, are thought to be important in the prevention of allergic diseases. When a baby is put into an incubator, his skin and gut are often colonized by bacteria different from his mother's and studies show that the baby is much more likely to adjust to his new world, metabolically speaking, when he is skin-to-skin with the mother than if he is in that incubator.

We now know that this is true not only for the baby born at term and in good health, but also for the premature baby. Skin-to-skin contact and Kangaroo Mother Care can contribute much to the care of the premature baby. Even babies on oxygen can be cared for skin-to-skin, and this helps reduce their need for oxygen and keeps them more stable in other ways as well.

From the point of view of breastfeeding, babies who are kept skin-to-skin with the mother immediately after birth for at least an hour are more likely to latch on without any help, and they are more likely to latch on *well*, especially if the mother did not receive medication during labor or birth. Putting mother and baby skin-to-skin can also be a valuable first step in solving any breastfeeding difficulties they are having.

To recap, skin-to-skin contact immediately after birth which lasts for at least an hour has the following positive effects on the baby. These babies:

- are more likely to latch on.
- are more likely to latch on well.
- have more stable and normal skin temperatures.
- have more stable and normal heart rates and blood pressures.
- have higher blood sugars.
- are less likely to cry.
- are more likely to breastfeed exclusively longer.

There is no reason that the vast majority of babies cannot be skin-to-skin with the mother immediately after birth for at least an hour. Hospital routines, such as weighing the baby, should not take precedence. Of course, there is also no reason a baby cannot be back skin-to-skin with the mother immediately after the hospital routines are done.

The baby should be dried off and put on the mother. Nobody should be pushing the baby to do anything; nobody should be trying to help the baby latch on during this time. The mother, of course, may make some attempts to help the baby, usually in response to the baby's behaviors showing some interest in going to the breast, and this should not be discouraged. The mother and baby should just be left in peace to enjoy each other's company. (The mother and baby should not be left alone, however, especially if the mother has received medication. It is important that not only the mother's partner, but also a nurse, midwife, doula, or physician stay with them—occasionally, some babies do need medical help and someone qualified should be there "just in case.") The eye drops and the injection of vitamin K can wait a couple of hours. By the way, immediate skin-to-skin contact can also be done after cesarean section, even while the mother is getting stitched up, unless there are medical reasons which prevent it.

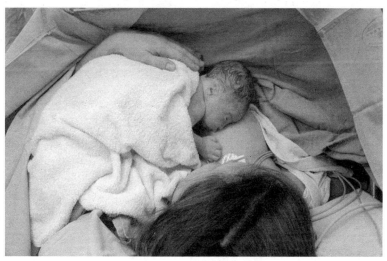

Skin-to-skin contact while mother is having her incision for caesarean section sewn up.

Studies have shown that even premature babies as small as 1200 g (2 lb 10 oz) are more stable metabolically (including the level of their blood sugars) and breathe better if they are skin-to-skin immediately after birth. The need for an intravenous infusion, oxygen therapy, or a nasogastric tube, for example, or all the preceding, does not preclude skin-to-skin contact. Skin-to-skin contact is quite compatible with other measures taken to keep the baby healthy. Of course, if the baby is quite sick, the baby's health must not be compromised, but any premature baby who is not suffering from respiratory distress syndrome can be skin-to-skin with the mother immediately after birth. Indeed, in the premature baby, as in the full term baby, skin-to-skin contact may decrease rapid breathing into the normal range.

Even if the baby does not latch on during the first hour or two, skin-to-skin contact is still good and important for the baby and the mother for all the other reasons mentioned.

I have heard of a few cases where a mother had planned not to breastfeed, but was still urged by hospital staff to hold her baby skin-to-skin. After doing this for a short period of time and seeing her baby gravitate to her breast, these mothers decided to breastfeed after all. The effects of this simple technique are powerful! In fact, one could say that skin-to-skin contact is even more important if the mother does not breastfeed so that the mother and baby have this special opportunity to "fall in love with each other."

References

Risks of Not Breastfeeding

Kallio MJT, Salmenperä L, Siimes MA, Perheentup J, Miettinen TA. Exclusive breastfeeding and weaning: effect on serum cholesterol and lipoprotein concentrations in infants during the first year of life. *Pediatrics* 1992;89:663-6.

Wingard DL, Criqui MH, Edelstein SL, Tucker J, Tomlinson-Keasey C, Schwartz JE, Friedman HS. Is breastfeeding in infancy associated with adult longevity? *Am J Pub Health* 1994;84:1458-62.

Joneja JMV. Breastmilk: a vital defence against infection. *Can Fam Phys* 1992;38:1849-55.

Yang KD, Bohnsack JF, Hill HR. Fibronectin in host defence: implications in the diagnosis, prophylaxis and therapy of infectious diseases. *Pediatr Infect Dis J* 1993;12:234-9.

Goldman AS. The immune system of human milk: antimicrobial, anti-inflammatory and immunomodulating properties. *Pediatr Infect Dis J* 1993;12:664-71.

Kunz C. Rudloff S. Biological functions of oligosaccharides in human milk. *Acta Paediatr* 1993;82:903-12.

Xanthou M, Bines J, Walker WA. Human milk and intestinal host defence in newborns: an update. *Advances in Pediatrics* 1995;42:171-208.

Hanson LÅ. Breastfeeding stimulates the infant immune system. *Science & Medicine* 1997;4:2-11.

Bernt KM, Walker WA. Human milk as a carrier of biochemical messages. *Acta Paediatr* 1999;Suppl 430:27-41.

Importance of Latch

Righard L, Alade MO. Sucking technique and its effect on success of breastfeeding. *Birth* 1992;19:185-9.

Effects of Labor Medications

Lie B, Juul J. Effect of epidural vs general anaesthetic on breastfeeding. *Acta Obstet Gynecol Scand* 1988;67:207-9.

Nissen E, Lilja G, Matthiesen AS, Ransjo-Arvidsson AB, Uvnas-Moberg K, Widstrom AM. Effect of maternal pethidine on infants' developing breastfeeding behaviour. *Acta Paediatr* 1995;84:140-5.

Winberg J. Examining breastfeeding performance: forgotten influencing factors. *Acta Paediatr* 1995;84:465-7.

Nissen E, Widstrom AM, Lilja G, Matthiesen AS, Uvnas-Moberg K, Jacobsson G, Boreus LO. Effects of routinely given pethidine during labour on infants' developing breastfeeding behaviour. Effects of dose—delivery time interval and various concentrations of pethidine/norpethidine in cord plasma. *Acta Paediatr* 1997;86:201-8.

Riordan J, Gross A, Angeron J, Krumwiede B, Melin J. The effect of labor pain relief medication on neonatal suckling and breastfeeding duration. *J Hum Lact* 2000;16:7-12.

Skin-to-Skin Contact

Mikiel-Kostyra K, Mazur J, Boltruszko I. Effect of early skin-to-skin contact after delivery on duration of breastfeeding: a prospective study. *Acta Paediatr* 2002;91:1301-6.

Christensson K. Fathers can effectively achieve heat conservation in healthy newborn infants. *Acta Paediatr* 1996;85:1354-60.

Christensson K, Bhat GJ, Amadi BC, Eriksson B, Höjer B. Randomised study of skin to skin versus incubator care for rewarming low risk hypothermic neonates. *Lancet* 1998;352:1115.

Williams AF. Hypoglycaemia of the newborn: a review of the literature. *World Health Organization*, Geneva. 1997.

Christensson K, Siles C, Moreno L, Belaustequi A, De La Fuente P, Lagercrantz H, Puyol P, Winberg J. Temperature, metabolic adaptation and crying in healthy fullterm newbornds cared for skin-to-skin or in a cot. *Acta Pediatr* 1992;81:488-93.

Jansson UM, Mustafa T, Khan MA, Lindblad BS, Widstrom AM. The effects of medically-oriented routines on prefeeding behaviour and body temperature in newborn infants. *J Trop Pediatr* 1995;41:360-3.

Rooming-In

McBryde A. Compulsory rooming-in in the ward and private newborn service at Duke Hospital. *J Am Med Assoc* 1951;145:625-8.

Yamauchi Y, Yamanouchi I. The relationship between rooming in/not rooming and breastfeeding variables. *Acta Paediatr Scand* 1990;79:1017-22.

Saadeh R, Akre J. Ten steps to successful breastfeeding: a summary of the rationale and scientific evidence. *Birth* 1996;23:154-60.

Risks of Artificial Nipples

Mizuno K, Ueda A. Changes in sucking performance from Nonnutritive sucking to Nutritive sucking during breast- and bottle-feeding. *Pediatr Res* 2006;59:728-31

Gomes CF, Trezza EMC, Murade ECM, Padovani CR. Surface electromyography of facial muscles during natural and artificial feeding of infants. *J Pediatr (Rio J)* 2006;82(2):103-9

Newman J. Breastfeeding problems associated with early introduction of bottles and pacifiers. *J Hum Lact* 1990;6:59-63.

Lang S, Lawrence CJ, L'E Orme, R. Cup feeding: an alternative method of infant feeding. *Arch Dis Child* 1994;71:365-9.

Armstrong H. Techniques of feeding infants: the Case for Cup Feeding. *Research in Action* 1998;no 8:1-6.

Howard CR, de Blieck EA, ten Hoopen CB, Howard FM, Lanphear BP, Lawrence RA. Physiologic stability of newborns during cup and bottle feeding. *Pediatrics* 1999;104:1204-7.

Malhotra N, Vishwambaran L, Sundaram KR, Narayanan I. A controlled trial of alternative methods of oral feeding in neonates. *Early Hum Dev* 1999;54:29-38.

Gupta A, Khanna K, Chattree S. Cup feeding: an alternative to bottle feeding in a neonatal intensive care unit. *J Trop Pediatr* 1999;45:108-110.

Kliethermes PA, Cross ML, Lanese MG, Johnson KM, Simon SD. Transitioning preterm infants with nasogastric tube supplementation: increased likelihood of breastfeeding. *JOGNN* 1999;28:264-73.

Righard L, Alade MO. Breastfeeding and the use of pacifiers. *Birth* 1997;24:116-20.

Barros FC, Victor CG, Semer TC, Filho ST, Tomasi E, Weiderpass E. Use of pacifiers is associated with decreased breastfeeding duration. *Pediatrics* 1995;4:497-99.

Aarts C, Hörnell A, Kylberg E, Hofvander Y, Gerbre-Medhin M. Breastfeeding patterns in relation to thumb sucking and pacifier use. *Pediatrics* 1999;104:e50.

Unrestricted Feeding

Illingworth RS, Stone DGH. Self-demand feeding in a maternity unit. *Lancet* 1952;April 5:683-87.

Salariya EM, Easton PM, Cater JI. Duration of breastfeeding after early initiation and frequent feeding. *Lancet* 1978;November 25:1141-43.

Lucas A, Lucas PJ, Baum JD. Differences in the pattern of milk intake between breast and bottle fed infants. *Early Hum Dev* 1981;5;195-99.

de Carvalho M, Robertson S, Friedman A, Klaus M. Effect of frequent breastfeeding on early milk production and infant weight gain. *Pediatrics* 1983;72:307-11.

Klaus MH. The frequency of suckling: a neglected but essential ingredient of breastfeeding. *Obstet Gynecol Clinics of North America* 1987;14:623-33.

Yamauchi Y, Yamanouchi I. Breastfeeding frequency during the first 24 hours after birth in fullterm neonates. *Pediatrics* 1990;86:171-5.

Avoiding Supplements

Shrago L. Glucose water supplementation of the breastfed infant during the first three days of life. *J Hum Lact* 1987;3:82-6.

Nylander G, Lindemann R, Helsing E, Bendvold E. Unsupplemented breastfeeding in the maternity ward: positive long term effects. *Acta Obstet Gynecol Scand* 1991;70:205-9.

Hill PD, Humenick SS, Brennan ML, Woolley D. Does early supplementation affect long-term breastfeeding? *Clinical Pediatrics* 1997;June:345-50.

Breastfeeding for Premature Babies

Hedberg Nyqvist K, Ewald U. Infant and maternal factors in the development of breastfeeding behaviour and breastfeeding outcome in preterm infants. *Acta Pædiatr* 1999;88:1194-1203 *(prematures can breastfeed)*.

Marinelli KA, Burke GS, Dodd VL. A comparison of the safety of cup feedings and bottle feedings in premature infants whose mothers intend to breastfeed. *J Perinatology* 2001;21:350-5 *(babies more likely to desaturate during bottle feedings compared to cup feedings)*.

Chan M, Nohara M, Chan BR, Curtis J, Chan GM. Lecithin decreases human milk fat loss during enteral pumping. *J Pediatr Gastroenterol Nutr* 2003;36:613-5.

O'Connor D, Jacobs J, Hall R, Adamkin D, Auestad N, *et al.* Growth and development of premature infants fed predominantly human milk, predominantly premature formula, or a combination of human milk and premature formula. *J Pediatr Gastroenterol Nutr* 2003;37:437-46.

Lubetsky R, Vasman N, Mimouni FB, Dollberg S. Energy expenditure in human milk versus formula fed preterm infants. *J Pediatr* 2003;143:750-3 *(human milk fed infants used less energy)*.

Collins CT, Ryan P, Crowther CA, McPhee AJ, Patterson S, Hiller JE. Effects of bottles, cups and dummies on breastfeeding in premature infants: a randomised controlled study. *Br Med J* 2004;329:193-8 *(prematures fed with cups rather than bottles were more likely to leave hospital breastfeeding)*.

What is a good latch and why is it important?

The definition of a good latch is very simple: a good latch is comfortable for the mother and allows the baby to get milk easily and well.

But *getting* that good latch is sometimes much more complicated, especially if the baby hasn't gotten off to the best start.

Babies feed quite differently at the breast than they do on a bottle. To start with, you can force the firm nipple into the baby's mouth even if he's not really interested. He doesn't have to open his mouth wide or take an active role in the process when he's given the bottle. With a bottle, the baby typically has the nipple only a short distance inside his mouth, even if the nipple is quite long. Milk will drip from the hole in the nipple into his mouth (especially if someone jiggles the bottle a little) and when he sucks, more milk will flow out. Often the baby uses his tongue to press up against the nipple to slow down the flow when he needs to take a breath. The firm rubber nipple pressing against his palate provides a strong stimulus to suck and the rapid flow of milk means he has to continue sucking or drown.

To get milk from the breast, the process is very different. The baby needs to participate much more actively. It's not possible to force the mother's nipple into the baby's mouth; he must open his mouth wide and actively take it in. He needs to take the nipple much further back in his mouth than if it was a bottle nipple, so that it rests against the soft palate rather than the hard palate. That means that a good portion of the breast will be in the baby's mouth as well. His tongue must go under the nipple and breast, cupping the breast and extending over the baby's bottom gums and lip. The baby holds the breast in place by sucking, but uses his tongue, moving in rhythmic waves, to squeeze the ducts in the breast and the movement of his lower jaw to compress the ducts further and transfer the milk into his mouth. The asymmetric latch is most effective in making this possible because it allows the baby's bottom jaw (the only one that moves) to cover a large area of the breast (and therefore more of the ducts) and the position encourages the baby to latch on with his tongue down and forward where it will naturally go under the breast.

Unlike formula, which is the same from the beginning of the feeding to the end, human milk changes throughout the feeding and from one feeding to another. A good latch is important throughout the entire feeding to ensure that the baby is getting the full range of milk, not just what pours out from the breast in the first few minutes with a mother whose milk is abundant. The idea that the milk changes from "foremilk" to "hindmilk" after a certain number of minutes is simply not true. The change is gradual, not abrupt, so there is no dividing line between foremilk and hindmilk. The exact composition of the milk depends on how recently the baby last nursed, the time of day, and other factors as well.

The rate of flow of the milk also changes throughout the feeding. At the beginning of the feeding after the first few seconds or minutes of the baby beginning to suckle, especially in the early weeks, the milk will "let down" and flow quickly – in fact, many mothers have a problem with milk leaking. Then, as the feeding continues, the flow normally slows down, meaning the baby depends less on the mother's milk ejection reflex to get milk and more on his own efforts.

A baby may have a poor latch and still be getting lots of milk, especially in the early days when most mothers have more than enough milk. However, if the poor latch continues, problems may emerge. The mother's nipples may get damaged and sore, and the milk supply may gradually decrease (see chapter 10 on Late Onset Slow Weight Gain). Once this starts to happen, the baby who has become used to the fast flow may pull off in frustration, leading to more nipple pain and increasing concerns about milk supply for the mother.

How can a mother get as good a latch as possible? It should be emphasized again that there are issues, both in babies and in mothers, which can prevent them from achieving the "perfect" latch, but the better the latch, the more milk the baby will get, and the less likely the mother is to get nipple soreness.

It is not absolutely essential for a baby to latch on using the techniques described for breastfeeding to go well. Indeed, since the majority of mothers are perfectly capable of producing more than enough milk for their babies, in many cases, almost any latch will do *if* the mother does not try to limit feedings in any way and if she is not bothered too much by nipple soreness. Nipple soreness, by the way, is not a given even with a poor latch. Nipple soreness almost always means the latch is poor; however, absence of nipple soreness does not mean the latch is good.

The worse the latch, however, the more the baby depends on the mother's milk ejection reflex (MER) in order to get milk. This will mean that even if the mother has an abundant supply, the feedings may be long or frequent, or both. Mothers may have several milk ejection reflexes during a single feeding, but they do not necessarily occur in rapid sequence. Thus, when the mother has an abundant supply, but the baby has a poor latch, the baby will drink when the flow is rapid (as during a milk ejection reflex, for example) and, especially during the first weeks, sleep or seem to sleep at the breast when the flow slows. If there is another MER, the baby will drink some more and continue to "hang out" at the breast waiting for more milk. The mother may feel that the baby nurses "continuously" or "all the time." In less industrialized societies, this is not considered to be a problem, it seems, and mothers will keep the baby at the breast for long periods of time and/or may return the baby to the breast very frequently. It has been reported that the women of the Bushmen in Southwest Africa often will put the baby to the breast 4 or more times an hour. Some mothers, even in North America, will report that they breastfeed 20, 30, or more times a day and are unconcerned about this frequency. They simply carry the babies with them and barely interrupt what they are doing as they offer the breast.

But that's certainly not the rule. Generally, in industrialized societies, and more and more amongst the affluent in less industrialized societies, babies are supposed to be "good" - meaning they feed only every 3 to 4 hours, or at most, every two hours (often because the mothers believe that otherwise the breast won't have a chance to "fill up"). And, of course, each feeding is expected to take at most perhaps 20 to 30 minutes. This "numbers" approach to breastfeeding is a disastrous way of thinking about breastfeeding and is ruining breastfeeding for many mothers (and babies).

However, health professionals in industrialized societies need to take into account this worry about babies feeding "too frequently or too long" on the breast. And the way to reduce this concern is to get the best latch possible, so that babies will be "more efficient" at breastfeeding and won't return to the breast so often or stay on the breast so long that the mothers get discouraged because the babies are not "following the rules." Of course, it's also important to remind mothers that babies nurse for many reasons besides eating. Breastfeeding is more than food. So, sometimes a baby with an excellent latch who is getting plenty of milk will still want to come to the breast frequently – for comfort, for reassurance, to help him fall asleep, to make him feel better when he's sick, etc.

Working with baby's cues

Babies are born with the skills and instincts to help them breastfeed, but we often ignore the messages and cues they are sending us. It is much easier to help a mother latch her baby on if the baby is calm yet ready to nurse. The entire process becomes far more difficult when the baby is upset, exhausted from crying, overly hungry, or not hungry at all. So it is valuable to tune into the baby's cues and internal rhythms so that breastfeeding happens when the baby is ready.

Help mothers to recognize the baby's early signs of wanting to nurse. If she is holding the baby skin-to-skin, the baby may move towards the breast on his own. Even without the skin-to-skin component, if she is holding the baby upright against her chest, he will signal his interest in feeding by shifting to one side and moving down her body into position to breastfeed. Some babies will almost throw themselves to the side in an attempt to get into position.

If the baby is sleeping in a separate bassinet or incubator, he may show his desire to nurse by smacking his lips and sticking his tongue out repeatedly, putting his fists to his mouth, squirming from side to side and opening his mouth, sucking on his fingers or the blanket, and other sometimes subtle behaviors. Help the mother to observe her baby and get to know his early cues. If she's not sure if the baby really wants to breastfeed, she can always try it and see. If he really doesn't want to eat, he won't. Waiting until the baby is crying is not helpful, as it makes learning to latch more difficult.

What does a good latch look like?

A baby who is well latched on has what I call an "asymmetric" latch. It is different from what has been taught for many years. I owe this "revolutionary insight" to Chloe Fisher and Anne Barnes who taught me how much difference this asymmetric latch makes when babies are put to the breast. I am not entirely sure why it works better, but I have no doubt that it does, and I wish to thank Chloe and Anne for their insights and keen sense of observation. Much of what we have learned about breastfeeding has come not from double blind randomly assigned studies (impossible in any case with regard to breastfeeding), but rather from people understanding breastfeeding, observing women and babies together as they breastfeed, and gaining yet more understanding from these observations.

When a baby is well latched on with this asymmetric latch, his chin touches the breast – in fact, is usually buried in the breast - but his nose does not touch the breast. (Only when the mother's breasts are extremely large, might the nose touch the breast, but even then, it usually will not.) He covers more of the mother's areola with his lower lip than his upper lip. The baby's lower lip is flanged outwards, not sucked in. If one looks at the baby's head from the mother's side, he is also slightly turned upward so the lower part of his body is slightly closer to the mother than the upper part. This too is different from the teaching of the last few years in which the baby is described as being "tummy to tummy" with the mother, meaning "flat" against the mother.

Getting the best latch possible

There are multiple ways of getting the baby onto the breast with the "ideal" latch. Indeed, I frequently see mothers doing absolutely nothing special, letting the baby grab the breast without any attempt by the mother to "get the baby on just right," and the baby takes the breast and looks exactly as he should. We also need to recognize that every mother-baby dyad is unique – in fact, the mother's two breasts will not be identical – so that sometimes the latch and the latching techniques benefit from some "fine-tuning."

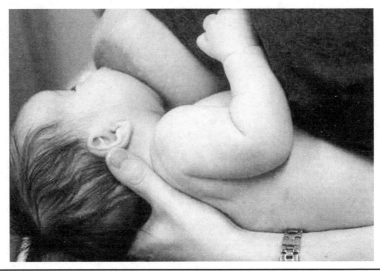

Note that the baby is in a straight line with his head slightly tilted backward. The mother is pushing in his bottom with her forearm, while her hand is palm up under his face (the web between thumb and index finger is in the nape of the baby's neck).

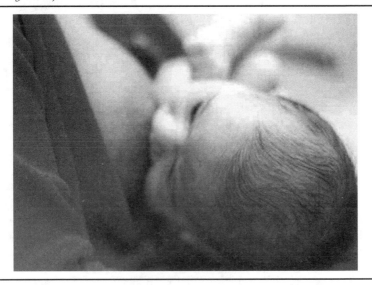

The baby is slightly tilted upward towards the mother.

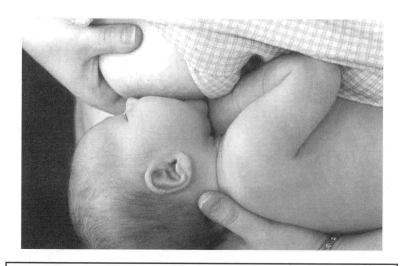

A "symmetric" latch. It works often enough, but when this photo was taken, the baby was hardly drinking any more at the breast. By asking the mother to push in the baby's bottom with her forearm, the baby swiveled a little, ended up with an asymmetric latch (without taking him off the breast), and he started drinking well again.

It is not uncommon, though, for women to experience difficulty positioning and latching the baby on. This may be in part because most of us see far more babies being fed out of bottles than babies at the breast. I see many mothers who are essentially and unconsciously imitating bottle-feeding positions and techniques when they try to put their babies to the breast.

The way I shall describe below is, in my opinion, the easiest way to do it and succeeds most of the time. Thus, differences between what I suggest and what others suggest may just be a difference in the way we think it is easiest, not really a fundamental difference. It can be worthwhile to have some other techniques "up your sleeve" as some mothers find some positions more comfortable, and sometimes an approach that works with one baby doesn't work as easily with another. The goal is not to be following a set of "rules" but to achieve an effective latch.

First, it is important to consider timing. Mothers need to be aware of the early feeding cues their baby shows – the baby sucking on hands in his sleep, smacking lips, restless, turning towards mother and rooting, etc. If she waits until the baby is crying, it will be harder to get a good latch. I still hear from many mothers that the nurses tell them to wait to feed until the baby is screaming because then his mouth is open wide! Sure, his mouth is open wide but his tongue is pulled up and he is likely to lunge or grab at the nipple as soon as it gets close. The baby needs to be calm – if the baby is screaming and frantic, it is better to help him calm down, perhaps by giving him a little milk in whatever way works, so that he'll be ready to go to the breast.

When the mother is sitting, I will usually suggest to her that she use the cross-cradle position to hold the baby. I find this position the easiest to get started with, but the same principles apply whether the baby and mother are lying down together, side by side, or if the mother uses the football hold, the "traditional" cradle hold, or the Madonna hold: the idea is still to get that asymmetric latch.

Proper positioning and latching

Getting the baby into a good position is essential for getting a good latch. For the purposes of explanation, let us assume that the mother is feeding on the left breast.

Good positioning facilitates a good latch. A lot of what follows under latching comes automatically if the baby is well positioned in the first place.

The Cross Cradle hold is often the easiest for teaching and for the mother to learn latching techniques because both you and she can see what the baby is doing and she has more control over the baby's head.

Undressing the baby down to just a diaper is often helpful in positioning as it allows mother and baby to be closer. If the mother is wearing a bra, it is often helpful to have her pull the entire cup below her breast or remove the bra during this learning stage.

Help the mother position the baby on her right arm, with the baby's bottom towards her elbow. She then uses the **side** of her forearm to push the baby's bottom close to her and turns her hand palm upwards (this should happen automatically, but mothers often have a tendency to rotate their elbows to hold the baby's shoulder, as they are frequently taught to do this), so that the baby's head is resting on her hand as if it were a pillow under his head. This will help her support the baby's body more easily and also bring the baby in from the correct direction so that he gets a good latch. The mother's hand will be palm up under the baby's head, and the web between her thumb and index finger should be **behind the nape of his neck** (not behind his head). The baby will be almost horizontal across the mother's body, with his head slightly tilted backward, and should be turned so that his chest, belly, and thighs are against the mother *with a slight tilt* so the baby is looking up. There should not be any space between the mother's body and the baby, and his bottom should be tucked in close to her.

You may want to use one or more pillows to help the mother maintain this position, especially if the baby is heavy.

Now have the mother support her left breast with her left hand. She can put her fingers against her ribcage under the breast and her thumb on the top of the breast. If her breasts are too large to do this comfortably, her fingers can support the bottom of the breast, but it is important to be sure they are well back from the nipple and areola.

The baby should be approaching the breast with the head *just slightly* tilted backwards and the nipple aimed towards his nose. The nipple then automatically points to the roof of the baby's mouth.

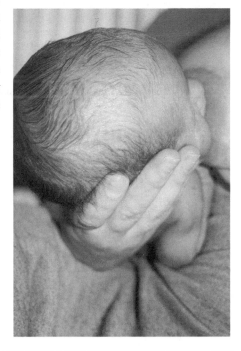

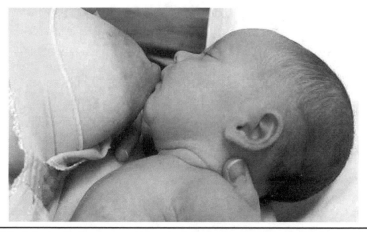

The baby is sleeping because he just had the first good feed in his life (because for the first time the mother was shown how to latch him on). The photo was staged to show the position of the baby with regard to the nipple (pointing to the roof of the baby's mouth, even to his nose).

Let's go through the sequence of the mother holding her baby with her right arm and offering her baby the left breast. Use the photos to help understand the description.

1. **The mother tucks the baby's bottom in closer to her with the *side* of her right forearm. Note the following points:**

    *   If the mother uses the side of her forearm, the palm of her hand faces upwards.

    *   The baby's weight is mainly on her forearm rather than on her hand or wrist.

    *   Pushing in the baby's bottom with her forearm is a key element in getting the baby to latch on with an *asymmetric latch*.

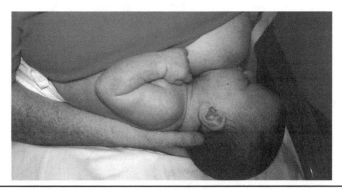

The mother pushes the baby's bottom in with the side of her forearm.

2. **The mother places her hand under the baby's face, almost as if her hand were a pillow for the baby. This allows the mother to support the baby's head and maintain the baby's going towards the breast at the "correct angle." Note the following:**

   - The mother will have her thumb on the upper side of the baby's head or neck, with the web space between the thumb and first finger directly in the nape of the baby's neck. She should not have her thumb as far forward as the baby's cheek as it is difficult to move the thumb that far forward, not because of concern of activating the rooting reflex.

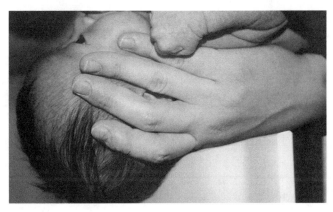

The mother's hand is palm up under the baby's face.

If the mother uses the above methods of holding the baby (the pushing in with the mother's forearm is very important), the baby will come towards the breast with the mother's nipple pointing to the roof of the baby's mouth. Now, the mother needs to get the baby to open his mouth **wide**. She can press into her breast slightly with her thumb to keep her nipple pointed towards the roof of the baby's mouth, and move the nipple lightly across the baby's upper lip, from one corner of the baby's mouth to the other. Another technique that may work is to have the mother start right at the bottom of baby's nose and stroke the nipple down that little groove between the nose and the mouth and onto the top lip. With the baby snuggled in well, the breast usually touches the bottom lip as well. Almost inevitably when the nipple is moved down from the nose to that top lip, the baby opens his mouth wide - and the nipple is in a perfect position, pointed towards the top of baby's mouth and you get a really nice asymmetrical latch. This works better than using the nipple to stroke the baby's lower lip. If she finds it difficult to do this, she might find it easier to use her other hand (the one supporting the baby) to move the baby so that his upper lip rubs against the nipple.

3. **The mother runs her nipple along the baby's upper lip (not lower), from one corner to the other, until the baby opens his mouth wide.**

   - The area representing the mouth on the sensory projection in the brain is very large and correspondingly very sensitive and usually results in the baby's opening wider than usual, often to the surprise of the mother.

   - It is for this reason that I believe the up and down "tickling" of the baby's lip (from nose to chin) does not work as well to get the baby to open his mouth wide as running the nipple along the baby's upper lip.

   - Furthermore, the up and down motion, from nose to chin and back, will often result in the baby's opening wide when the nipple is pointing to the lower part of the baby's mouth, which results in the latch being less good.

4. **Wait for the baby to open up as if yawning.** If his head is tipped slightly back as we've described, his tongue should naturally fall to the bottom of his mouth, ready for the breast to go on top of it. Once the baby opens his mouth wide, the mother brings the baby *straight* onto the breast, with a brisk movement of her whole arm, remembering to keep some pressure pushing the baby's bottom into her own body. As the mother brings the baby toward the breast, his **chin** should touch the breast first. She shouldn't push his head forward or scoop him around so that the nipple points to the middle of his mouth; she needs to maintain the angle so that the nipple is still pointing to the roof of his mouth.

   - *Straight* onto the breast means the baby will actually touch the breast first with his chin, and his nose will probably not touch the breast at all.

   - Curling the baby around, so that the nipple ends up in the middle of the baby's mouth and both the nose and chin touch the breast results in a latch that is not as good. This can happen if, for example, the mother's hand is higher up on the baby's head, so she pushes his head towards the breast with her hand, rather than using her whole arm to move the baby in.

5. **Thus, once the baby is on the breast well, the "latch" looks as follows:**

   - The baby's chin touches or is buried in the breast.

   - The baby's nose does not touch the breast. Even when the mother has very large breasts, it is unusual for the baby's nose to touch the breast if he is well latched on.

   - The baby's lower lip is flanged outward. So is the upper lip, though I am not convinced that the upper lip being flanged is of as much importance.

   - The baby covers more of the areola with his lower lip than with his upper lip.

   - The baby's whole body is slightly tilted upwards.

   - The baby's mouth is wide open.

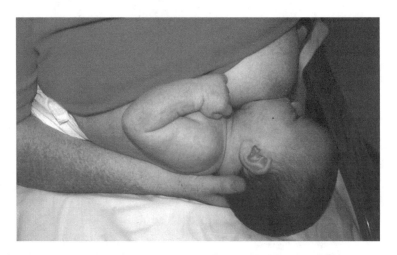

The "big picture." True the baby's neck could be a little more extended, but first comfortable feeding for this mother.

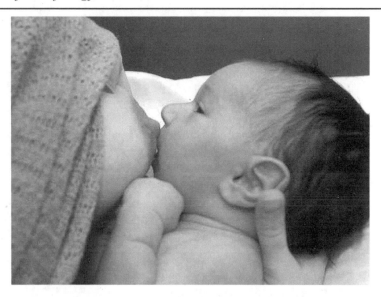

Mother tickles the baby's upper lip with the end of her nipple, lightly, tickling only, from one corner of the mouth to the other. Note mother's hand position. Left hand well placed on breast, right hand well placed on baby. The mother is not pointing the nipple to the roof of the mouth. This happens automatically.

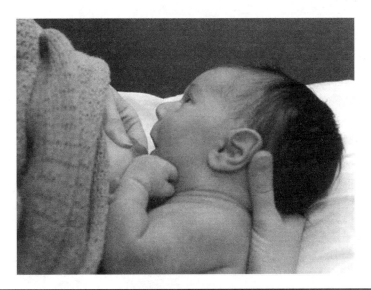

Baby opens mouth wide, but puts hand in way to frustrate photographer. Somehow mother has slipped hand down on the breast. Not a good idea, as it will be difficult for the baby to get a good mouthful of breast.

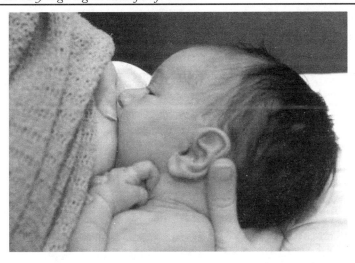

Mother brings baby onto the breast, not breast into baby's mouth. Almost latched on. Note that there is always the same relationship between the baby's head and the mother's breast (no bringing the baby up and around, but rather straight onto the breast). Mother's hand is still too close, however.

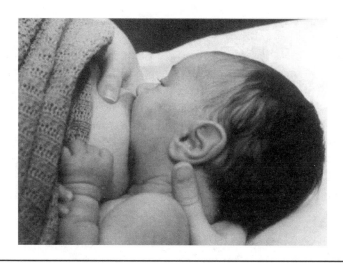

Well latched on. Chin in breast, but not the nose. The baby covers more of the areola with his lower lip than his upper.

If the baby's lower lip is not flanged outward, the mother or helper can pull the lower lip out by putting some mild downward pressure on the baby's chin. This does not take a lot of force. You are really only holding down the chin. Usually, the mouth will open wider and the lower lip will flange outwards. In theory, it should not be necessary to do this; in practice, especially if the baby has had bottles, it may be very helpful.

It is not always easy to achieve the "ideal" latch. Babies latch on better when there is more milk. There will be more milk when the baby latches on well and breastfeeds well. Because the baby will get more milk if he is latched on well, he will help the mother produce more milk if he draws more milk out of the breast. Thus, there is a potential vicious circle that is set up if the above does not happen, and a nice circle if it does. Waiting too long to achieve the "ideal" latch may result in the milk supply decreasing. With a decreasing milk supply, the baby may latch on less well, resulting in his drawing less milk out of the breast and the milk supply decreasing even more.

A slightly different approach that is sometimes useful, especially with babies who resist the breast altogether and with babies who have become used to taking bottles so that as soon as the nipple touches their lip they grab for it and try to suck it in like a bottle nipple, is described below.

With this approach, the mother keeps the hand supporting the baby below the baby's head and behind just the neck and shoulders. (This is helpful for babies who have been repeatedly forced onto the breast and have come to strongly resist the feeling of a hand on the back of their heads.) The baby's head will tip back. The mother positions the baby so that her nipple is level with the baby's nose, and brings the baby in close so that she touches his mouth with the curved area of her breast below the nipple. The feel of that rounded breast against his mouth will usually cause the baby to open his mouth very wide (and there is no nipple for him to grab!); as he does so, the mother can use one finger or her thumb to press down on her breast and help the nipple go under his top lip (if necessary). This results in an asymmetric latch.

Wait and watch

If the mother complains that latching the baby on is painful, try to make some adjustments without removing the baby. Remember that it is a very short distance between a painful latch and a comfortable one, so you may be able to shift the baby enough to relieve her discomfort. The baby's lower lip may be rolled in, and you may be able to use your finger (or have the mother use hers) to gently hold the chin down so that it is flanged out against the breast. Try making the latch more asymmetrical by letting the baby's head tip back a bit more while tucking his bottom in close. Sometimes using breast compression to get some milk flowing will encourage the baby to give some good, deep sucks, and this helps pull the nipple into a better position.

Do not tell mothers to take the baby on and off the breast several times to get the perfect latch. If the baby goes on and off the breast 5 times and it hurts each time, the mother will have 5 times more pain, and worse, 5 times more damage, and a frustrated baby and a frustrated mother. It is better to adjust the latch a bit while the baby is at the breast, often by having the mother push in a bit with her elbow and forearm. Improve the latching-on technique a bit more when putting him to the other breast, or at the next feeding.

The same principles apply whether you are sitting or lying down with the baby or using the football hold. Get the baby to open wide; don't let the baby latch onto the nipple, but get as much of the areola (brown part of breast) into the mouth as possible (not necessarily the whole areola).

Football hold

In this position, the mother sits upright with her baby at her side. She may need to sit near the front of the chair, with pillows supporting her back, so that the baby can't push his feet against the back of the chair. To feed the baby on her left breast, she lays the baby on his back on her left forearm and supports her breast with her right hand, with her fingers well back from the areola. Her left hand is under the lower part of the baby's head, with the web between her thumb and first finger behind the baby's head. The exact position she uses will depend on the size and shape of her breasts. (Note in the diagram at the end of this chapter that the baby could be going to the breast in the football hold or lying down, for that matter—the principles are the same no matter which way the baby is held).

The mother needs to position the baby so that her nipple is level with the baby's nose and his chin is close to the breast. He will be looking up towards her. As she runs the nipple along the baby's upper lip from one corner of his mouth to the other, he will open his mouth wide, and the mother then uses her whole arm, keeping the baby tucked in and close to her body, to bring him onto the breast. Using her whole arm to bring the baby on is important. Mothers often swivel the baby's head onto the breast using their wrists, but this results in a more "symmetric" latch. There is a tendency to do this even more with the football hold than with the cross cradle hold.

This position is helpful for women who have had cesarean births and who find it painful to have the baby against their abdomens. However, the cross cradle hold also works because the baby is held horizontally and is usually fairly far from the mother's incision. The football hold is often helpful with small premature babies and with babies who have come to resist the more common positions for breastfeeding because they have been repeatedly forced to the breast in those positions. It may also be helpful for the mother with large, soft breasts. But a baby who latches well with the football hold should be able to latch well with any hold. I am not a fan of the football hold because it is too easy to latch the baby on poorly as many mothers bend the baby's neck as he comes on to the breast resulting in a symmetric latch.

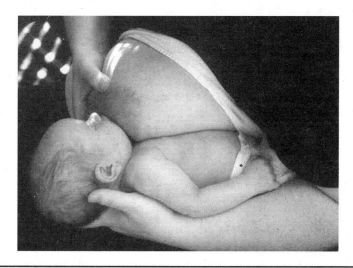

Football hold (this is the mother's right breast). The baby's neck could be a little more extended, but at least he has an asymmetric latch. Too many babies latched on in the football hold do not.

Side-lying

I think it is valuable for all mothers to learn to breastfeed lying down as it helps them get more rest. This position is also helpful for women with cesarean incisions or painful stitches that make it difficult and uncomfortable for them to sit up. It also can be good for women with large breasts because in this position they don't have to support the full weight of their breasts and may find it easier to see what the baby is doing.

To feed on the left breast, have the mother lie down on her left side. She may need pillows to help support her, especially if she has had a cesarean birth. (At home, she might find it helpful to have her partner lie behind her to support her.) She should also have pillows under her head to raise it up so she can see what she's doing, and so she doesn't have to use her left hand and arm to support her own head. The baby should be positioned on his side, with the nipple level with his nose and his lower body angled in towards his mother's body. If her breasts are very small, you may need to use a flat, firm pillow to elevate the baby so that he is level with the mother's nipple.

When the baby is first learning this position, the mother may find it easiest to roll slightly back, using her left hand to support her breast and positioning her right hand behind the baby's neck, shoulders, and head, with her right forearm behind the baby's back . As before, the mother runs her nipple along the baby's top lip and moves him in close once his mouth is open wide so that he will latch on.

Once the baby gets good at this, mothers often switch hands so that her left hand is behind the baby's head, neck, and shoulders and her right hand supports her breast.

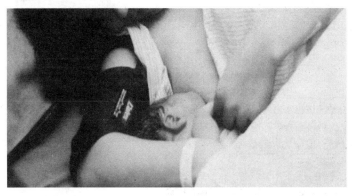

Sidelying immediately after birth. Looks exhausting, right?

Cradle hold

This is the traditional position seen in paintings of the Madonna and child around the world.

The mother who is using the cross-cradle position can change to this position once the baby is latched on well and nursing comfortably. She just moves the hand that was supporting her breast and puts that arm under the baby's body, then her other hand is free to take a drink of water, hug her toddler, or provide support to her breast if needed.

To initiate a feeding in this position, the baby lies on the mother's left arm to go to the left breast, with his head near her elbow and his bottom supported by her hand. His head will not be in the crook of her arm but rather on her forearm and will be allowed to tip back, with his neck and shoulders supported by her forearm. As before, he is rolled slightly onto his back so he is looking up towards his mother and the breast. Her right hand supports her breast and helps to aim the nipple towards his nose. When his top lip is stroked from one corner of the mouth to the other and he opens his mouth wide, the mother brings him in close, using her hand to tuck his bottom in close to her body.

The mother's posture

In any of these positions, it's important to make sure the mother is comfortable. If the mother is leaning forward, hunched over, or straining to support her baby's weight, she's going to be in some pain, sooner or later. Often she will unconsciously shift her position and the latch will deteriorate as the baby can no longer get a big mouthful of breast.

Nursing pillows are often recommended to prevent these problems, but many of these are not well designed and may not fit the individual mother. Help her find an arrangement of pillows that helps her sit comfortably and supports the arm that is holding the baby's weight. A book or footstool under her feet can also make a big difference in terms of her comfort.

Improving the baby's suckle

The baby learns to suckle properly by nursing and getting milk into his mouth. The baby's suckle may be made ineffective or not appropriate for breastfeeding by the early use of artificial nipples or from poor latching on from the beginning. Some babies just seem to take their time developing an effective suckle. Suck training and/or finger feeding may help, but note, taking the baby off the breast to finger feed is not a good idea and should be done as a last resort only. Really, babies learn to breastfeed by breastfeeding.

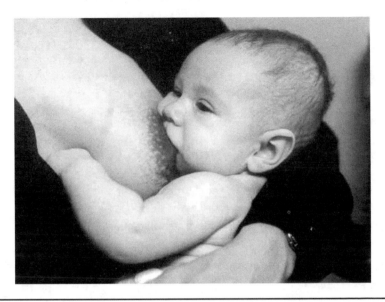

Poor latch. This 4-month-old is only 1 kg (2.2 lb) above birth weight. Her older brother gained very well exclusively breastfeeding.

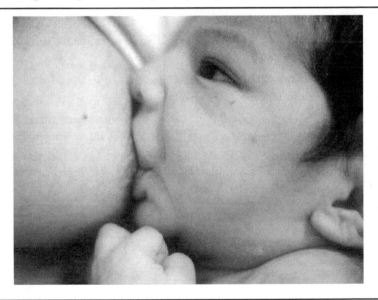

Poor latch. Baby is 2 weeks old, not gaining in spite of a mother's abundant milk supply.

LATCHING: SUMMARY FOR PARENTS

- Push baby's bottom into your body with the side (the side where your baby finger is) of your forearm. This will bring him towards your breast with the nipple pointing to the roof of his mouth.

- The mother's hand should be under the baby's face, palm up.

- Support head but DO NOT push in against breast.

- The baby's head will be tilted, almost automatically, slightly back.

- Wrap baby's body and legs in around mother.

- The baby will come to the breast, his chin will touch the breast first. The nose should usually not touch the breast.

- Use your whole arm to bring baby onto the breast, when baby's mouth is open wide.

- WATCH LOWER LIP, aim it as far from the base of the nipple as possible, so tongue draws lots of breast into mouth.

- Move baby's body and head together – keep baby uncurled.

- Make sure top lip is close to nipple, areola should show above lip when baby is latched.

- Keep chin close against breast.

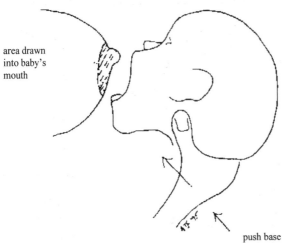

area drawn
into baby's
mouth

push base of hand firmly
against baby's shoulders
keeping baby " uncurled "
chin coming in first

WIDE MOUTH

Need mouth wide before baby is moved onto breast. Teach baby to open wide by:

- moving baby toward breast, touch top lip against nipple.

- moving mouth away SLIGHTLY.

- touching top lip against nipple again, move away again.

- repeating until baby opens wide and has tongue forward.

- Or, better yet, running nipple along the baby's upper lip, from one corner to the other, lightly, until baby opens wide.

MOTHER'S VIEW WHILE LATCHING BABY

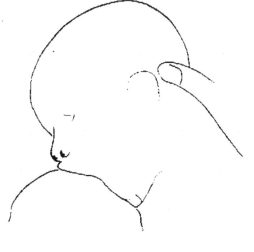

baby's head tilted
slightly back

bring baby in
quickly

push with base of
hand on
shoulders

area baby
draws in
mouth

chin touches first

baby's body
close against
mother

Move baby not breast

MOTHER'S VIEW OF NURSING BABY

head tilted slightly
back

chin well in against
breast

hold in firmly
against shoulders
keeping baby
uncurled

Diagrams by Anne Barnes

RECOMMENDATIONS FOR THE MOTHER

Mother's posture

- sit with straight, well-supported back
- face her trunk forwards, lap flat

Baby's position before feed begins

- place on pillow - can be helpful
- point nipple to baby's upper lip or nostril

Baby's body

- placed not quite tummy to tummy, but slightly on his back so that baby comes up to breast from *below* and baby's eyes make contact with mother's

Support breast

- raise breast slightly with fingers placed flat on chest wall below the breast, thumb is on top of the breast pointing up to firm inner breast tissue (if helpful, also use sling or tensor bandage around breast)

Move baby quickly onto breast

- tilt head back slightly
- push in across shoulders so chin and lower jaw make first contact (not nose) while mouth still wide open
- keep baby uncurled
- aim lower lip as far from nipple as possible so baby's tongue draws in maximum amount of breast tissue

CAUTIONS

Mother needs to AVOID:

- pushing her breast across her body

- chasing the baby with her breast

- flapping the breast up and down

- holding breast with scissor grip

- not supporting breast

- twisting her body towards the baby instead of slightly away

- aiming nipple to center of baby's mouth

- pulling baby's chin down to open mouth

- flexing baby's head when bringing to breast

- moving breast into baby's mouth instead of bringing baby to breast

- moving baby onto breast without a wide open mouth

- not moving baby onto breast quickly enough when baby opens mouth wide

- having baby's nose touch breast first and not the chin

- holding breast away from baby's nose with a finger (not necessary if the baby is well latched on as the nose will be away from the breast anyway)

References

Aldrich CA, Hewitt ES. A self-regulating feeding program for infants. *J Am Med Assoc* 1947;135:340-2.

McNeilly AS, McNeilly JR. Spontaneous milk ejection during lactation and its possible relevance to success of breastfeeding. *Br Med J* 1978;2:466-8.

Howie PW, Houston MJ, Cook A, Smart L, McArdle T, McNeilly AS. How long should a breastfeed last? *Early Hum Dev* 1981;5:71-7.

Woolridge MW, Ingram JC, Baum JD. Do changes in pattern of breast usage alter the baby's nutrient intake? *Lancet* 1990;336:395-7.

Dewey KG, Heinig J, Nommsen MS, Lonnerdal B. Maternal versus infant factors related to breastmilk intake and residual milk volume: the DARLING study. *Pediatrics* 1991;87:829-37.

Tyson J, Burchfield J, Sentence F, Mize C, Uauy R, Eastburn J. Adaptation of feeding to a low fat yield in breastmilk. *Pediatrics* 1992;89:215-20.

Righard L, Flodmark C-E, Lothe L, Jakobsson I. Breastfeeding patterns: comparing the effects on infant behavior and maternal satisfaction of using one or two breasts. *Birth* 1993;20:182-5.

Colley JRT, Creamer B. Sucking and swallowing in infants. *Br Med J* 1958;August 16:422-3.

Drewett RF, Woolridge M. Sucking patterns of human babies on the breast. *Early Hum Dev* 1979;3/4:315-20.

Woolridge MW, Baum JD, Drewett RF. Effect of a traditional and of a new nipple shield on sucking patterns and milk flow. *Early Hum Dev* 1980;4/4:357-64.

Woolridge MW, Baum JD, Drewett RF. Does a change in the composition of human milk affect sucking patterns and milk intake? *Lancet* 1980;December 13, 1980:1292-3.

Pollitt E, Consolazio B, Goodkin F. Changes in nutritive sucking during a feed in two day and thirty day old infants. *Early Hum Dev* 1981;5:201-10.

Drewett RF. Returning to the suckled breast: a further test of Hall's hypothesis. *Early Hum Dev* 1982;6:161-3.

Nysenbaum AN, Smart JL. Sucking behaviour and milk intake of neonates in relation to milk fat content. *Early Hum Dev* 1982;6:205-13.

Marmet C, Shell E. Training neonates to suck correctly. *MCN* 1984;9:401-7.

Smith WL, Erenberg A, Nowak A, Franken EA. Physiology of sucking in the normal term infant using realtime US. *Radiology* 1985;156:379-81.

Woolridge MW. The 'anatomy' of infant sucking. *Midwifery* 1986;2:164-71.

McBride MC. Sucking disorders in neurologically impaired infants: Assessment and facilitation of breastfeeding. *Clinics in Perinatology* 1987;14:109-31.

Marchini G, Lagercrantz H, Feuerberg Y, Winberg J, Uvnäs-Moberg K. The effect of non nutritive sucking on plasma insulin, gastrin and somatostatin levels in infants. *Acta Pediatr Scand* 1987;76:573-8.

Maher SM. An overview of solutions to breastfeeding and sucking problems. *LLL International* revised 1988.

Assessing the Latch

Whenever a breastfed baby is seen by a health care professional, a feeding should be observed, especially in the first few weeks. This is as basic and given the errors that are often made when weighing babies, especially when different scales are compared, more crucial than weighing the baby. It should be as routine as listening to the baby's heart. If there are any concerns about breastfeeding, weight gain, complaints of nipple or breast pain by the mother, then observing the baby at the breast in order to assess the latch and other aspects of the feeding is the best way of making a diagnosis of what has gone wrong.

During the newborn stage, careful assessment of the first feedings is very important for many reasons: to prevent (or fix) nipple damage, to ensure the baby is getting as much of the milk as possible, to establish milk production, to provide teaching for the new mother at an important stage so that she can continue to get a good latch, and to decrease the "need" for supplementation (which should be rarely necessary and increases the risk of early weaning). Assessment at this stage is intended primarily to prevent problems. But problems often arise from the very first feeding, so assessment can show us the way to fix problems, too. It also provides a unique opportunity at this point to help the mother understand what constitutes a good latch, and more importantly, teach her how to know a baby is getting milk. Once the mother knows that the "pause in the chin" means "I just got milk," the mother can cut through so much of the poor information about breastfeeding that is out there. For example, the still heard "feed the baby 20 minutes on each side" loses any credibility once the mother knows how to tell if the baby is getting milk. A baby who feeds really well for 20 minutes, say, on the first side may not take the second. A baby who "nibbles" at the breast for 20 hours may still not get enough.

After the first few days, an assessment is most often needed as part of the investigation of a problem, but still can be preventative, too. For example, a mother may bring in a baby for a routine check believing that everything is hunky-dory because the baby falls asleep at the breast. She mistakenly interprets the sleepiness as a sign of the baby's contentment, but in fact the baby is not really feeding well, is not getting much milk, and responds as many babies do to slow flow by falling asleep (as is often seen when a baby is given a pacifier). Observing a feeding and assessing the latch at this point can catch a problem before it turns into a disaster.

Some concerns that might arise that may be related to latch include: baby may not be gaining weight appropriately, the mother may be experiencing nipple pain, or the mother may have concerns about the frequency and/or length of the baby's feedings. This may have been a problem since the beginning or may have begun suddenly (perhaps after the baby has been given some bottles, for example). In these situations, the assessment is intended to offer clues as to the possible causes of the problem so that solutions can be found.

The latch cannot be assessed from the doorway of the room while the mother sits in bed or on a chair breastfeeding. And it cannot be assessed by a two-second glance at the mother while she feeds the baby. On the other hand, it does not require a 40 minute observation period either. A few minutes are usually sufficient, in conjunction with the history, to give a good idea of what's going on.

Step One: Listen to the mother

Ask the mother how it feels when the baby is nursing from beginning to end. When the baby is feeding well, **she should not feel pain** from the baby's suckling. (In the first few days, mild tenderness is perhaps "normal," but it should be mild and decreasing by the 3rd or 4th day after birth.) If the mother does describe pain, you want to know when and where it hurts. Some mothers feel the sensation of the milk letting down through the ducts (which can be quite strong and may be described as painful, although, usually only for the first few days or at most a few weeks). Others will describe burning nipple pain or shooting pains in the breast, which are often due to a Candidal infection and not due primarily to a poor latch, though a damaged nipple sets the stage for a Candidal infection (recommendations for dealing with these problems are discussed elsewhere). The mother may feel some discomfort, tugging or pressure as the baby latches on, but her nipples should not hurt or be blistered or damaged.

Even if the latch "looks good" and even if the baby seems to be getting some milk or even plenty of milk, it is a problem if the mother is experiencing pain. It means something is wrong. Pain is a signal, a message, not a normal part of breastfeeding. Some women have so much milk in the early weeks that it doesn't matter how badly the baby is latched, he'll be getting milk – it just flows into his mouth. You'll notice that if the baby lets go of the nipple for a second, the milk will spray all over. But despite this rapid flow of milk, if the latch is not good, the mother may be in significant pain.

What the latch looks like from the outside is not the only thing that matters. The movements of the baby's tongue and jaw must also be correct in order for the baby to get milk and for the mother to feel comfortable as the baby nurses.

Sometimes mothers are told that if breastfeeding hurts for the first minute or so (or the first thirty seconds, or until she counts to one hundred), but improves after that, then things are fine. This is not true. It usually means that the baby is not latched on deeply enough at first, but that he then tugs the nipple into the correct position as he sucks. It can be because the mother isn't waiting for the baby to open his mouth wide enough, or because her fingers are in the way when he goes to latch on at first, or because of the position she's holding the baby, or because the baby has had some bottles and so expects to use suction to pull the nipple in.

This pattern of initial pain followed by decreasing pain is also sometimes seen in a baby with a tongue-tie, who will rub against the nipple at first with his tongue, then if the milk begins to flow quickly as it lets down, will stop moving his tongue and the pain subsides. In this case, however, the mother often experiences another bout of nipple pain when the letdown of milk slows and the feeding continues.

A considerable amount of damage can be done to the nipple in that first minute (repeated 8, 10, 12, or more times a day), and over time many mothers find that the feedings become more and more painful throughout because the nipple is bruised, blistered, and cracked.

Some babies will pull their tongues back in their mouths as they nurse and use the back of their tongues to press up against the nipple. This sometimes happens with babies who have been given bottles - to slow or stop the flow of milk from a bottle nipple, the baby needs to push up on the bottle nipple with his tongue. When the baby goes to the breast again, he may try to do the same thing – and it hurts! Some babies who have never had bottles or pacifiers may also start doing this if their mothers have milk that flows very rapidly (sometimes called over-active letdown). It's a way of trying to reduce the amount of milk that is coming.

A tight frenulum that restricts the movement of the tongue may also make the baby rub the mother's nipple with his tongue because the baby is not able to extend his tongue and cup the breast the way he is supposed to. The baby ends up trying to move his tongue up and down to extract the milk, causing this kind of pain.

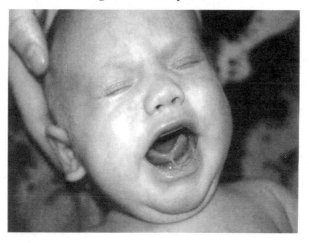

Obvious tight frenulum. Though the baby is crying, he cannot lift his tongue as babies do when they cry. He also cannot use his tongue properly when breastfeeding.

When the nipple does not go far enough into the baby's mouth, he is "nipple-feeding" (or worse, nipple sucking only without feeding) instead of "breast-feeding." Instead of the nipple being at the back of the baby's mouth where the tissue is soft and protects the nipple, and the suction created is spread over the entire surface of the nipple, the nipple is usually being compressed between the baby's tongue and hard palate. Only a small part of the nipple is exposed to the stripping action of the baby's tongue against the palate. When the nipple comes out of baby's mouth, you will usually see that the shape is distorted (it looks like a new lipstick) and there is often a line of blistering or damage across the middle or lower edge of the nipple.

This can be caused by a tongue-tie if the baby is pushing up with his tongue or by a positioning problem if the nipple is not being placed far enough back in the baby's mouth.

It is only a very short distance between a position that puts the nipple between the tongue and hard palate creating severe pain and a position that puts the nipple against the baby's soft palate where it is comfortable and feedings are painless. Just moving the nipple half an inch or even a quarter of an inch (50 to 100 mm) deeper into the baby's mouth can make all the difference in the world.

Sometimes mothers describe the baby clamping down on the nipple and bruising her. Often, if you watch the baby you will see that she is quite right – the baby does indeed seem to bite down on the breast or nipple repeatedly.

This can happen with a baby who is tongue-tied or unable to extend his tongue properly. He may try to compensate for not being able to extract milk the usual way by trying to compress the nipple and breast. Babies who are not deeply latched on may also do this in an attempt to get the milk to flow; babies also sometimes do this to slow down the milk when it is coming too quickly, especially if they've had some bottles and have used this approach to stop the flow of milk from the bottle nipple.

Babies often clamp down when they aren't getting a good flow of milk and a vicious cycle results – the baby is not latched on well, doesn't get much milk, clamps down, gets less milk, and so on.

The opposite of clamping down is the baby who repeatedly slips off the nipple. He sucks for a time, then slips off. Sometimes he then "grabs" for the nipple or lunges at it with his mouth – creating a painful moment for the mother. When a baby is well latched on, the nipple is securely and deeply in his mouth. Babies do not normally easily slip off the breast – in fact, you usually have to get a finger in the baby's mouth almost forcefully if you want to break the suction! Sometimes when you watch these "slipping off" babies, you see that the nipple is just barely in the baby's mouth.

This behavior is sometimes seen in babies as a result of medication during labor and birth. They may have difficulty coordinating sucking during the first few days or weeks due to the side effects of the medication, and often when the nipple is in their mouths they don't seem to know what to do with it. They may not suck at all or may suck for a few seconds then slip off the nipple.

In other cases, the baby simply has not gotten a deep enough latch to stimulate the baby's suckling. If you put your finger in a baby's mouth, you'll notice that some will start sucking strongly even when your finger is near the front of their mouth. For others, they need to feel that stimulation near the back of the mouth to get them suckling properly. When the breast is not deeply in the baby's mouth, they suck half-heartedly and will slip off easily.

Sometimes when mothers have a very rapid milk flow and a generous milk supply, the baby will suck this way to minimize the milk flow so he's not choking and drowning! These babies quickly learn that they can just hold the nipple in their mouths and the milk will arrive with little or no effort on their part. While this works for a while, it may become a problem because it can cause sore nipples. Even if the mother's nipples are not damaged, difficulties may result later when the mother's milk production slows down and the baby doesn't know how to extract milk effectively. In these situations, it is helpful to take steps to reduce the milk flow to a level that is more manageable for the baby while improving the latch.

Some pain may not be related to latch.

While most often pain while nursing is caused by latch difficulties, there are other possible causes. Sometimes mothers describe **burning pain** in their nipples that continues between feedings as well as during the feeding. This is often due to an infection with *Candida albicans*, commonly known as thrush, though "thrush" properly speaking, applies only to the white patches in the baby's mouth (see photo).

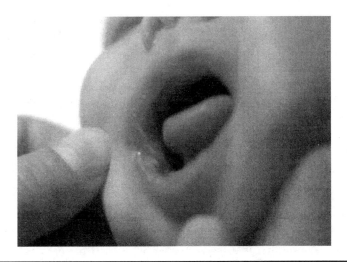

Thrush in the baby's mouth. In fact, the mother attended the clinic for reasons other than sore nipples, which she did not have. Note the tongue is not affected, as it usually is not. The presence of thrush in the baby's mouth does not mean the mother will have sore nipples, and its absence does not rule out a Candidal infection in the mother. If the mother is pain free and the baby is not bothered by his thrush, I usually do not encourage the mother to treat the thrush.

It's also important to note that a mother may not feel any pain, and yet the latch is not good and is not effective at extracting milk. Pain-free nursing does not guarantee that all is well.

Step Two: Observe the baby at the breast

Ask the mother to feed the baby the way she normally would. As you watch the baby nurse, here are some things to look for:

How is the baby positioned relative to the mother's body? Because most women see far more babies getting bottles than babies at the breast, many mothers hold their babies in a bottle-feeding position, then try to breastfeed them.

Common mistakes:

- The baby is lying on his back with his side against his mother rather than turned towards her.

- The baby is lying so that his head is well over to the side of the mother, resting in the crook of the mother's arm. This results in the baby getting a symmetric latch, or often, if the baby is quite far to the side, a "reverse" asymmetric latch with more of the areola covered by the baby's upper lip than the lower lip, instead of the other way around. (Refer to photo of the 4-month-old who has gained only 1 kg since birth on page 38.)

- The baby's head is near the mother's breast, but the rest of his body is angled away from the mother, rather than tucked in close to her. Usually this results in the baby's neck being bent and the chin not resting against the breast so that the baby won't open his mouth.

- The mother is using a nursing pillow, and the baby is lying on his back on the pillow or has rolled into the crack between the pillow and his mother. The result is she brings the breast to the baby - thinking the baby has to stay on the pillow - and not the baby to the breast.

- The baby is below the level of the breast so that the mother has to lean forward to bring her nipple to the baby's mouth.

As an aside, this is one reason that it can be very helpful for pregnant women to attend La Leche League meetings. At those meetings, they see many different women breastfeeding their babies and they learn – often quite unconsciously – how to hold a baby at the breast. It's a way to counteract the millions of images of bottlefed babies that most women have seen by the time they have their own babies.

Where are the mother's hands? Typically, a mother will use one hand to support her baby and the other to support her breast.

Probably the most important thing to remember about the hand supporting the baby is that it **must not be behind the top of the baby's head**. This is a very common mistake, but can create very significant problems when latching the baby on. For one thing, many babies will resist pressure against the back of their heads by pushing back and away from the breast. Some newborns seem to be unusually sensitive to pressure on their heads, so they will cry and try to escape the pressure if the mother pushes on their heads to get them to the breast. (See photo of the 4-month-old who has gained only 1kg since birth, page 38.)

Secondly, when mothers try to bring their babies to the breast with a hand behind the head, they almost always end up going "nose first." The nose is buried in the breast and the result is a shallow latch.

The supporting hand should, instead, be palm up underneath the baby's face, like a pillow under the side of his head. This allows the baby to come to the breast "chin-first" rather than "nose-first" with his neck slightly extended (head tipped back somewhat). With her hand in this position, the mother can more securely support the baby's entire body with her forearm and elbow. Babies need this feeling of being securely held to enable them to relax and nurse well. Mothers also feel more secure this way.

The position of the hand supporting the mother's breast is also important. Most mothers tend to focus on their fingers (or thumb) on the top of the breast while forgetting about where their fingers are underneath the breast. Often, their fingers are barely behind the nipple, making it impossible for the baby to get a good mouthful of breast. Mothers can be advised to put their hands against their ribs below the breast, then just bring their fingers out enough to provide some support to the breast. This helps to remind them how far back their fingers should be. Also, this hand position can be used to direct the nipple position, pointing up to the baby's nose, especially in women with large soft breasts. Normally, though, by putting pressure on the baby's bottom with the side of her forearm, the mother ensures that the baby will come at the breast at the right angle, and the nipple will be pointing to the roof of the baby's mouth.

Watch how the baby latches on to the breast. Is he grabbing at the nipple with his mouth only partially open? Is the mother attempting to feed the nipple into the baby's mouth like she would a bottle nipple? Does the baby latch on "chin-first," "nose-first," or straight down the middle? The asymmetric "chin-first" latch is much more effective.

What do you see when the baby is latched on well? His head should be tipped back so that he can look up at his mother. There should be a space between his nose and the breast. From the side, you may not be able to see his mouth at all because it is hidden by the curve of the breast. If you can see it, his mouth is clearly open very wide. His body is close to his mother and wrapped around her.

As the baby begins to nurse, observe how the baby suckles. When the baby is sucking properly and getting milk, you may initially see a series of rapid sucks, with baby's mouth opening and then closing again quickly. This is to stimulate the flow of milk. As the milk begins to flow, you will see slower sucks, with a pause in the movement of the chin when the baby's mouth is wide open. This pause is very important – it lets you know that the baby is getting a mouthful of milk. You or your patients can see this pause on video clips (as well as how to latch a baby on and more) at the websites www.breastfeedingonline.com, www.thebirthden. com/Newman.html or www.gentlemothering.ca amongst others. *Dr. Jack Newman's Visual Guide to Breastfeeding* DVD also shows these various techniques.

Does he seem to have only the nipple in his mouth and is making a rapid series of sucks, pausing occasionally with his mouth closed to rest? This baby is not latched deeply enough and will not be getting much milk.

Does he move back and forth on the nipple, letting it slip almost out of his mouth at times? This baby also doesn't have a good latch.

Do you hear clicking noises (mothers sometimes mistake this for swallowing sounds)? This usually indicates that the baby doesn't have a good seal and the "click" is the result of air getting into the baby's mouth with each suck –something that doesn't happen with a good latch.

Does the baby make short, fast sucks for a minute or two, then fall asleep – even though he seemed very hungry when he went to the breast? This is one of the behaviors that often confuses mothers. They assume that the baby was not really hungry because he falls asleep. But this is a baby who is giving up on breastfeeding and trying to conserve energy because he isn't getting any milk. If you can improve the latch and the baby's milk intake, you will usually see a dramatic change in behavior.

You may also see this in a baby who is responding to the flow of milk – when the milk flows quickly, he drinks, but as soon as it slows down, he drifts off to sleep, temporarily pacified but not really satisfied.

Even if the mother is not feeling any soreness, these are signs that the latch is not good and the baby may not be getting much milk. The way to know if the baby is getting milk, though, is to observe the way the baby sucks at the breast (see page 56, regarding the "pause").

At the same time, observe the **mother's responses.** Sometimes a mother will say that the latch is not painful (perhaps because she's heard that breastfeeding should not be painful or because she's afraid that she'll be told to wean if she admits that it hurts), but her body language makes it clear that it really hurts. She may wince or grimace as the baby latches on, but relax and talk in a normal voice as the feeding continues. Or she may sit tensely and obviously in pain through the whole feeding.

Step Three: Observe the breast and the baby at the end of the feeding

When either the baby lets go or the mother breaks the suction with her finger and removes the baby from the breast, it can be very helpful to observe the nipple as it emerges from the baby's mouth.

If the nipple is cylindrical in shape and slightly elongated, with no signs of damage, this is a sign of a good latch. (Although if the mother is in pain, the latch still needs work, regardless of the nipple's appearance.)

If the nipple is shaped like a new lipstick or a wedge with one side straight and the other slanted, the nipple is not going far enough back in the baby's mouth and is being compressed between baby's tongue and hard palate with just the tip at the soft palate. You may see a line of blisters or cracked or damaged skin at the thin edge that is exposed to the suction. This is sometimes seen in a baby with a tongue-tie.

If the nipple is flattened, it is not going very far into the baby's mouth, and the entire nipple is being compressed between the tongue and hard palate. You may see damage (blisters, cracks, bleeding) on the end of the nipple, and you may also see some bruising and sometimes cracking at the base of the nipple if the baby is also clamping down to hold the nipple in place.

If the nipple looks abraded or raw, it may be because the baby is tongue-tied and has restricted tongue movement or because the baby is using his tongue to stop the flow of milk.

If the nipple looks very pink and shiny, the mother may have a Candidal infection on her nipples. Sometimes you also see flaking skin on the nipples and areola with this condition. The mother may have a Candidal infection of the nipples without any visible signs of thrush in the baby's mouth. The mother may also have no visible signs on her nipples and still have an infection with Candida. An infection with Candida albicans will also cause nipple pain, usually described by the mother as burning or shooting pain.

Also observe the baby. The baby who has fed well looks relaxed, content, and satiated – like a "drunken sailor." But be careful in making assumptions about feeding based just on this, especially in the first few days to first week. Some babies fall asleep at the breast and don't wake up when they hardly get any milk. This is the baby who is at risk of becoming dehydrated, but becomes more wakeful and active when fed more. A baby who feeds well and sleeps, that's good. A baby who feeds poorly and sleeps, that's bad. In the latter situation, the baby does not necessarily need to be supplemented; often, fixing the latch is all that is necessary.

If the mother found the feeding painful, even if the baby seems very content, the latch still needs work – many babies will get enough milk in the early weeks just by opening their mouths and letting the milk pour in.

However, if the latch is not improved, the mother may wean because of the pain or her milk supply may drop over time because the baby doesn't know how to stimulate further milk production. So while a satisfied baby is a good sign, it does not necessarily mean all is well with the latch – just like a mother who is pain free does not mean the latch is good. You need both elements to be there.

The baby who is not getting enough milk will often have a worried expression on his face; even if he falls asleep he may bring his hands to his face or continue rooting for the breast. It is possible in this case that the baby is latched on well, but the mother is not producing enough milk;

however, it's most helpful to first check all aspects of the latch to ensure that it is as good as it can be before trying other steps to increase milk production.

Your observations during these stages of the feedings will help to reveal whether or not there is a problem with the latch and give you some ideas about fixing it.

And a reminder: if the mother is in pain and you notice that the latch is not good, it is not helpful to take the baby off, put him back on, take him off, put him back to the breast, over and over. Each latch tends to cause more pain, more nipple damage, and lots of frustration for the baby. Often small adjustments can be made while the baby is nursing which can make the feeding more comfortable. If one attempt to improve the latch doesn't work, let the baby finish the feeding and work on latching better next time.

References

Smith WL, Erenberg A, Nowak A, Franken EA. Physiology of sucking in the normal term infant using realtime US. *Radiology* 1985;156:379-81.

Woolridge MW. The 'anatomy' of infant sucking. *Midwifery* 1986;2:164-71.

Riordan J, Gill-Hopple K, Angeron J. Indicators of effective breastfeeding and estimates of breast milk intake. *J Hum Lact.* 2005 Nov;21(4):406-12.

Weigert EM, Giugliani ER, Franca MC et al. The influence of breastfeeding technique on the frequencies of exclusive breastfeeding and nipple trauma in the first month of lactation. *J Pediatr (Rio J).* 2005 Jul-Aug;81(4): 310-6.

Haughwout JC, Eglash AR, Plane MB, Mundt MP, Fleming MF. Improving residents' breastfeeding assessment skills: a problem-based workshop. *Fam Pract.* 2000 Dec;17(6):541-6.

4 Causes of Latch Problems

In our clinic population, we see many babies, presumably normal in every other way, who cannot latch onto the breast. This is very strange and puzzling. Why would a normal, healthy, full term baby not latch on well or not latch on at all? A baby who cannot breastfeed well would be in great danger in the hunter-gatherer society of our ancestors, and the ability of babies to latch on well to the breast would be a highly conserved evolutionary trait. Of course, some babies have obvious causes and these will be discussed further on. Interestingly, such babies who latch on poorly, or not at all, usually manage to take a cup, finger feed, or bottle feed just fine. It seems that we are interfering with the baby in some way with the result that the baby does not latch on to the breast well.

What has gone wrong here? Infants are normally born with the instincts and abilities to breastfeed, but from there on it becomes a learning process, like walking, learning to ride a bicycle, or learning to talk. Like these processes, the breastfeeding skill is enhanced and reinforced by doing. In other words, babies learn to breastfeed *by breastfeeding*. Anything that interferes with their breastfeeding may result in their not learning how to breastfeed properly.

While babies learn to breastfeed by breastfeeding, breasts are often making milk in abundance. During the early postpartum period, babies can still gain well, even without the baby latching on well. In many such cases, the milk essentially falls into the baby's mouth without the baby really breastfeeding well, so the baby gains weight. However, in the longer term, the mother's milk supply may diminish when the baby does not breastfeed well, resulting eventually (by 3 or 4 months after birth) in the baby no longer gaining well, even after an initial rapid weight gain.

Birthing practices

Over the past few years, it has become increasingly obvious that many of the practices we have adopted around labor and birth have resulted in babies not breastfeeding well. Many such practices were adopted to make labor and birth "easier" for women, but were usually adopted in the era when breastfeeding and the behavior of the baby at the breast were not taken into account. Indeed, few studies were designed to evaluate possible effects of the intervention or medication on the mother and even fewer on the baby. Perhaps, not so co-incidentally, the rise in interventions in childbirth paralleled the decline in breastfeeding. As more and more health professionals and especially lactation consultants have begun asking questions about why a normal baby would not take the breast well or why a normal baby would have sucking problems, attention to birthing practices is providing at least some of the answers.

There is no question that fewer and fewer women in industrialized societies are having normal births. In many North American hospitals, 90% or more of women in labor receive epidural anesthesia. In some, cesarean section rates are over 30%. Despite lack of evidence of benefit, electronic fetal monitoring is widespread. Induction of labor is similarly almost routine, with many babies being born at "near-term" (37 or 38 weeks).

Many physicians will argue that the interventions are often necessary, preventing morbidity in the mother and/or baby, and saving lives. Of course, nobody will deny that interventions are *sometimes* necessary and even lifesaving, but they are not necessary as often as they are being used. Studies in the early 1990's showed us that many of the interventions that are commonly used during labor and birth are much less likely to be necessary if the mother gets good support during labor. For example, Kennel and Klaus in 1991 published a study that compared the rates of interventions during labor in three different groups of laboring women. In one group, each woman was supported during labor by a trained doula. In the second group, another woman, not trained to support labor, was in the room with the laboring woman. In the third group, the control, the laboring woman did not get any special support, a situation unfortunately all too common in industrialized countries. What were the results? In the doula-supported group of 212 women, the rate of epidural anesthesia was about 8%, whereas in the group of 204 women with no special support, it was 55%. The women in the group who had an untrained woman with them had an intermediate rate of epidural anesthesia of about 23%. In fact, for all the following interventions, the results were similar: the rate of oxytocin augmentation of labor, the rate of cesarean section, and even the rate of forceps delivery. Furthermore, the rate of sepsis evaluation of the newborn was lower in the supported group as well. More recent studies have shown that epidural analgesia in itself causes fever in the mother, and as a corollary, results in more frequent sepsis evaluation of the baby. *And, finally, the mothers were more likely to be successful at breastfeeding.* This is true even if the doulas have no particular training or interest in breastfeeding. The significant point here is that these medical interventions, each of which carries known risks to mother and/or baby, can be avoided by something as simple as having a support person present with the mother. These interventions undoubtedly interfere with the baby's being able to breastfeed well.

Electronic fetal monitoring

In a survey of mothers delivering between 2000 and 2002, 93% had electronic fetal monitoring. This is quite amazing for a technique for which there is no evidence of benefit to mother or baby. Health professionals insist on "evidence-based" medicine, except when it comes to what they do.

This technique requires a mother to be lying down (actually, it is possible with some advanced technology to allow laboring women to walk around a bit, but most hospitals do not have it available, and it is often discouraged even when it is available). The problem with lying down to labor is that the mother cannot find a position of comfort. For some women, during some parts of labor, it *may* be lying down, but not for most women most of the time. Women in labor who are allowed to move around freely will discover positions that make them more comfortable, and these change as the labor progresses and the baby's position shifts. Walking during labor has been shown to promote shorter labors with fewer interventions. Without this freedom to move around and find the most comfortable position, women often need more pain-relieving medications and perhaps augmentation of labor.

A review of studies involving 58,000 women in labor, looking at electronic fetal monitoring, showed that compared to the old technique of just listening to the baby's heart with a fetoscope, electronic fetal monitoring did not prevent perinatal death rates or lower Apgar scores. On the other hand, in all studies included, the rate of instrumental delivery and cesarean section was increased in the electronic fetal monitoring group.

Intravenous fluids

In the same survey, 86% of the women had received intravenous fluids during labor. Intravenous fluids are given as a routine, when the woman in labor has an epidural, for example, and is obligatory, obviously, if labor is augmented with oxytocin. This is considered a pretty benign intervention, and it has not been obvious to many that receiving intravenous fluids in labor may cause difficulties with breastfeeding.

In fact, receiving intravenous fluids may interfere in several ways. Again, because she is hooked up to an intravenous bag and often confined to bed (although the bag of intravenous fluid can be attached to a moveable pole so the mother can walk, this is still cumbersome), the mother may not be able to find a comfortable position so the risk of other interventions and instrumental delivery increases. Whatever makes labor and birth more difficult also makes breastfeeding more difficult.

However, there are other issues as well. For example, although this has not yet been demonstrated by research, it is likely that if the mother receives a liter or two of fluid over a relatively short period of time, she will experience increased fluid retention as will her baby. This is particularly true if she receives it in conjunction with synthetic oxytocin, which is an anti-diuretic hormone. This has two potential side effects.

In the mother: Lactation consultants have noted for years mothers having generalized edema after delivery, which also resulted in edema of the areola and nipple, making it difficult for the baby to latch on. When a baby has difficulty latching on, interventions, often inappropriate interventions such as giving bottles, are initiated and the baby's initial problems may be made worse.

In the baby: The results are somewhat more indirect. If the mother has fluid retention, there is no reason to believe that the baby will not also be born with extra fluid on board. What does this have to do with anything? Well, it has now become the "standard of treatment" that babies can only lose 10% of their birthweight during the first few days after birth (some say 7%, some even 5%). In many institutions, this has become a rule that is "carved in stone": "If the baby loses more than 10% or 7% or 5%, the baby must be supplemented." There is no scientific evidence to support this. In fact, one study found that breastfed babies who were supplemented with water or formula during the first few days lost *more* weight and were slower to regain the weight.

The fact that most babies are weighed on two different scales, which makes comparison of the two weights absurd, does not diminish the focus on weight loss or the rush to supplement. Helping the baby get more milk by fixing the breastfeeding (better latch on, use of compression to get the colostrum flowing, switching breasts when the flow slows, not limiting feeding times on the breast) is often ignored in the headlong rush to give supplementation.

Because in most hospitals, supplementation is given without fixing the way the baby latches on and is often given by bottle, the latch often becomes worse, potentially leading to problems later on. In other words we have "fixed" a problem in the short term, but not dealt with the real issues. In fact, the problem hasn't been fixed, only one of the symptoms has been fixed, which may or may not be significant. We have not done anything about the true problem, which is that the baby is not breastfeeding well. The minor initial problem may then become a long term problem. The interpretation will then be that the supplementation was a "marker" of difficulties rather than a partial cause of the difficulties.

Email received (2005): This is typical of many I have received, and I know this is what is happening in many postpartum areas.

- *"Within 36 hours of his birth, he had lost 9% of his weight – a fact which threw the nurses on the labor ward into a panicked flurry of activity. Within minutes of having weighed him, I was hooked up to a breast pump and being shown how to use the feeding tubes and syringe to supplement my baby with formula."*

Another email (2005): And there are long term consequences as well – the baby this mother is writing about is four months old:

- *"Think I got off to a bad start...the nurse told me.. [my baby] was losing too much weight (not even 10 percent of her birth weight in hindsight) and told me to get pumping. I have been worried ever since."*

So what does this mean in relationship to the baby whose mother is given IV fluids during labor? Well, this baby may be born with additional fluid in his or her system as a result, leading to an inflated birth weight. When the extra fluid is eliminated in the first day or two after birth, the baby's weight will be seen to have dropped significantly – perhaps below the "critical" (actually meaningless) percentage for supplementation.

Epidural anesthesia

When a mother is having an epidural (or spinal) anesthesia, she requires an intravenous infusion as well because the procedure is sometimes associated with a drop in blood pressure, and it is handy to have access to a vein. Having an epidural also inhibits the mother from walking around and finding a position of comfort. After all, it's not easy to walk around or get on hands and knees or squat when you cannot feel your legs.

But the epidural can cause other problems as well. In a study in 1997, Lieberman *et al* found that women who had epidurals during labor often had a fever as well, ranging from 7 or 8% with an epidurals for 6 to 12 hours to over 30% with an epidural for more than 18 hours.

In what way does this affect breastfeeding? If a woman in labor has a fever, she has tachycardia. And often, so does the baby. A baby with tachycardia may be in distress (it may be the fever, but we are not sure, better not take any chances), so interventions click in, interventions such as fetal scalp monitoring and scalp pH. Does the concern of the staff translate into anxiety in the mother? Of course it does, and anxiety in the mother is a well known inhibitor to the progression of labor. So labor may slow or even stop, and the risk of instrumental or operative delivery increases. The mother's intravenous infusion rate is upped to make up for increased fluid loss associated with fever, and the mother may receive antibiotics. In addition, when the baby is born, he is usually separated from the mother, a sepsis evaluation is made, often with blood counts, blood culture, even lumbar puncture, and the baby is given antibiotics. The initiation of breastfeeding is delayed. Babies learn to breastfeed by breastfeeding, but this baby born of a mother with fever during labor will not have a chance to begin breastfeeding for several hours, perhaps even a day or two (though such long separations are not at all necessary). Even though everyone knows, deep down, that the fever is caused by the epidural and the baby is fine.

In yet another study, the authors showed that epidural anesthesia is associated with a greater incidence of occiput posterior position at birth. And what happens when a baby is occiput posterior at birth? There is a lower chance of spontaneous vaginal delivery (only 25% of babies who are occiput posterior experience this kind of birth, compared to 75% of babies who are occiput anterior), the mother has a greater chance of having a significant perineal tear with a higher risk of postnatal wound infection, and the baby is more likely to have a lower 1 minute Apgar score. All these results have, as a corollary, the likelihood that the baby will be separated from the mother for variable periods of time ("no skin-to-skin contact until we repair this tear," for example, though why repair of the tear requires no skin-to-skin contact is beyond me).

Whatever controversies there may be about the risks of the use of epidural anesthesia, the studies are in agreement about three things. The use of epidural anesthesia is associated with:

1. an increased risk of maternal fever during labor.

2. an increased risk of instrumental delivery.

3. a longer second stage of labor.

All of the above may result in the baby and the mother being separated at birth for various reasons. For example, a prolonged second stage of labor is also associated with greater maternal fatigue. A common response of nursing staff to this situation is: "We'll take the baby away so you can get some rest."

Episiotomy

One of the most commonly performed interventions is the episiotomy. For years it was touted as the answer to preventing serious perineal tears in the mother and of helping the baby be delivered more easily and more rapidly. It has done none of these things, and happily, the rate of episiotomy is decreasing as birth attendants realize that the evidence is just not there to justify its use routinely. In fact, mothers often have increased pain because of the episiotomy, wound infection is not rare, and less rapid healing occurs than with a natural tear. In a recent meta-analysis in which studies compared "routine" episiotomy to "restricted use" episiotomy (where episiotomy was done only for definite indications), the authors concluded that there was no benefit to routine episiotomy, that "we identified fair to good evidence suggesting that immediate outcomes following routine use are no better than those of restricted use," and that "...routine use is harmful to the degree that some proportion of women...would have had lesser injury instead of a surgical incision."

Episiotomy, in itself, should not interfere with breastfeeding success, but in fact, all of the above mentioned difficulties (increased pain, increased use of antibiotics, etc.) interfere with the baby breastfeeding early and effectively because of the discomfort of the mother. The mother may find it difficult to sit up comfortably, for example. Somebody may even tell the mother that she cannot breastfeed if she is taking antibiotics (wrong 99.9% of the time).

Narcotic medication

In addition to other forms of analgesia, narcotics during and after labor may interfere with breastfeeding. It is obvious that a woman under the influence of narcotics may feel "out-of-control" and cannot react appropriately to her baby. In addition, the baby often cannot react appropriately to his mother, or anyone else for that matter. Studies going back many years have shown that babies influenced by maternal narcotics may have central nervous system dysfunction for many days, which may interfere with how they breastfeed. Meperidine (Demerol), having a long half-life, with an active metabolite that also has a long half-life, may affect a baby for a particularly long time. When babies do not suck properly or well, interventions are often brought into play that make breastfeeding success even less likely (trying to force babies to the breast and introduction of artificial nipples, for example).

Cesarean Section

Cesarean section, in effect, combines all the preceding impediments to getting babies to breastfeed early, latch on well, and breastfeed effectively. In the first place, all mothers who are going for cesarean section will have an intravenous infusion as well as anesthesia, --general, epidural or spinal, and in some situations local. There is no evidence for local anesthesia causing difficulties with breastfeeding, but there is with the other more commonly used methods.

Cesarean section is also associated with more problems with the baby, such as transient tachypnea, which often, according to hospital policy, requires separation of the mother and the baby. However, it should be noted that babies who are placed skin-to-skin with the mother immediately after birth have lower respiratory rates than if they are put into an incubator.

Finally, mothers who have had a cesarean section are in pain and require analgesia, often narcotic analgesia, with all the problems resulting from that. They very frequently have difficulty finding a comfortable position to breastfeed.

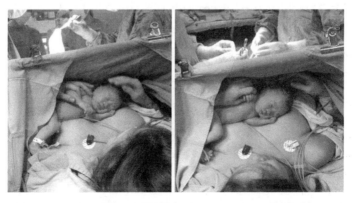

Skin-to-skin immediately after cesarean section, while the mother's incision is sewn up. Why cannot this be done everywhere? Because "we don't have c allow it."- Not good enough.

Separation of mother and baby

For generations now, we have been making excuses about why mothers and babies need to be separated after birth. Separation at birth often meant, at best, giving the baby a pacifier, or more likely, feeding the baby off the breast, usually with a bottle, which interfered with the baby latching on. The excuses were legion, and now most have been shown to be invalid. Here are just some of the reasons:

- The mother should rest after the baby is born. **Fact: Studies show the mother is better rested when she has the baby with her.**

- After a cesarean section, the baby and mother need to be separated. **Fact: Nonsense.**

- The baby needs to be observed by nurses in the hospital nursery after the birth, just in case. **Fact: There is no better observer of the newborn baby than his own mother.**

- Certain babies need treatment for low blood sugar. **Fact: Although this is true in some cases, the best way to prevent low blood sugar in the majority of babies is early skin-to-skin contact and early breastfeeding.**

- Babies who pass meconium *in utero* need to be observed. **Fact: The baby who is in trouble from meconium aspiration is in trouble immediately after birth and almost never in trouble after the first few minutes.**

- Premature babies need to be in special care. **Fact: Some do need specific medical interventions, but the bigger premature babies – the majority - are often better off with their mothers. Even tiny premature babies are better off in Kangaroo Care (skin-to-skin care) with their mothers.**

- If the mother is sick, it is better if the baby is not with her. **Fact: Obviously, if the mother is so ill that she is physically incapable of holding her baby, this is one thing, but the fact that she has a fever, a rash (with few exceptions), or a cough, etc., is not a reason to separate mother and baby.**

Actually, we now have evidence that most babies, particularly those who have not had exposure to central nervous system drugs during labor and birth, will often take the breast without any help, crawling up from the mother's abdomen and latching on all by themselves. When the baby does this, the latch is usually a good one – and the mother is greatly encouraged by seeing that the baby has done it all by himself. This should not be surprising, really. All newborn mammals in the wild must find the breast and latch on, and they need to be able to do it without the presence of a lactation consultant or a nurse; otherwise, they will die. Some mother mammals will instinctively guide the newborn towards the teat, but essentially the baby does it on his own.

So why does it seem so unusual for human babies to do the same thing? Well, if the mother is on the birthing table and the baby is across the room under the warming lamp, it would take a baby of considerably more advanced development than a newborn to find the breast. The mother and baby need to be in contact, skin-to-skin, and time needs to be given the baby to find the breast – not the ten minutes many hospitals allow for "bonding." Studies show that it takes, on average, about 50 minutes for the baby to find the breast and latch on all by himself. Even in those facilities that "allow" skin-to-skin contact immediately after the birth, it is rare that the baby stays with the mother for a full hour or two. Of course, the baby should stay there until he sleeps or finds the breast, even if finding the breast takes him 75 or 90 minutes. And really, is there any good reason to take the baby away after that? If we could keep mothers and babies together continuously from birth – not just in the same room, but in constant skin-to-skin contact - our breastfeeding problems would be significantly reduced.

Forcing a baby to take the breast

This is surely one of the major reasons babies do not latch on well, or even more commonly, refuse to take the breast at all. Hospitals tend to have a whole host of rules about infant feeding that don't match the reality of breastfeeding. Some have the notion that babies must feed every "x" hours – every three hours is the most common one – and if the baby doesn't take the breast at that point, "alternate feeding methods" are mandated. This often begins as early as three hours after birth. At the other end of the spectrum is the baby who wants to nurse very frequently in the early days – more often than every two hours.

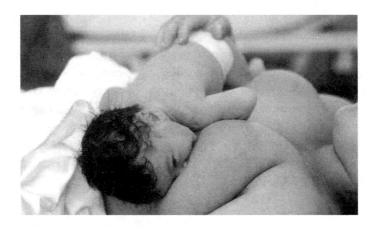

This baby is less than 90 minutes old (Note his hair is still wet). He has just crawled up to the breast and latched on by himself. In spite of the mother's large breasts. In spite of the mother's so called "flat nipples." (I think only in our bottle feeding mentality society would we call what most women have "flat nipples" because they don't look like bottle nipples.)

This is frequently taken as an indication that the baby isn't getting enough milk, and once again "alternate feeding methods" are introduced.

This is bad policy, often put into action by hospital staff who are poorly trained in helping mothers breastfeed. There is no evidence that babies must feed every three hours, not only in the first few days but also at any time. Babies who feed well will feed again when they are ready. In the first few days, babies have extra fluid on board, often obviating the "need" to feed frequently. Babies may want to feed frequently for a variety of reasons – including for comfort. Neither situation indicates an urgent need for supplementation.

Sometimes, in order to avoid supplementation, nurses will attempt to force the baby onto the breast. They help the mother position the baby, wait until the baby's mouth is open reasonably wide (often the baby is crying), and then rapidly push the baby's head towards the nipple. If the baby doesn't latch (the usual result), the nurse repeats the process. Sometimes they will hold the crying baby's head in place and instruct the mother to express some milk into the baby's mouth.

Anyone watching this process can see that it is clearly unpleasant for the baby. The baby pushes back against the nurse's hand or turns his head from side to side to evade the pressure. Because he's crying, his tongue is up near the roof of his mouth and an effective latch is almost impossible. Not only does he not latch on, he learns that being at the breast is an unpleasant experience. Often these babies will begin to cry as soon as they are held anywhere near the breast in anticipation of being forced once again.

Nipple and Breast Problems

Nipples come in many variations. Nipples can be large, they can be rather flat, and they can be inverted. But none of these types of nipples are abnormal and none should make a good latch impossible. They may in some cases make achieving a good latch more difficult, but not impossible. Often, the difficulty arises from the fact that the person helping the mother is simply unskilled at helping mothers.

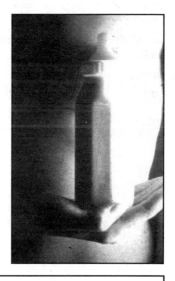

Most so-called flat nipples are actually quite normal. Unfortunately, too often we get our ideas of what a normal nipple on the breast is supposed to look like by what is called a nipple on the end of a bottle. The bottle nipple is long and rigid. This would not be a normal nipple if it were on the end of a mother's breast, but unfortunately we live in a culture where bottles are "normal" feeding devices for babies not breasts, so a woman with a normal nipple is thought to have flat nipples. If the baby has difficulty latching on, the nipple is often blamed.

I have seen 20,000+ women in our clinic for breastfeeding problems over the years. That's 40,000 nipples and I've never seen one woman's nipples shaped like this.

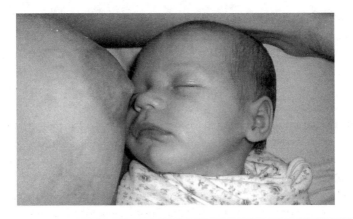

Photo sent as an example of a flat nipple. No, normal.

Breasts can come in all sorts of shapes and sizes, too. Very large breasts, especially if they are soft, may result in the mother's having difficulty latching a baby on, but this is due primarily to the difficulty in manipulating the breast and the baby, a mechanical problem, rather than some intrinsic problem with large breasts. In such cases, persistence and a little creativity often result in the baby's getting a good latch. For example, a sling, as used for supporting a broken arm, can be used to support the breast so that the mother has two free hands to latch the baby on. Some mothers with very large breasts find it easier, with a little help, to latch the baby on while they are lying down facing the baby. It sometimes helps to have the breast supported on a pillow.

It is vital when confronted with a baby who has difficulty latching on or latching on well to keep in mind that nipples and breasts change, and so do babies, and what is not possible on the first day of life, may very well be possible on the third day or the 10th day. One must not assume that if the baby cannot latch on well or at all today, that all hope is gone. Without hope, many mothers will give up breastfeeding, and that would be a shame.

We call it "breastfeeding" and not "nipple feeding" for a reason – the baby latches on to the breast and not just the nipple. The main difficulty with a small, flat nipple is that the baby may take the nipple into his mouth, but not feel the sensation against the top of his mouth and palate that stimulates him to begin sucking. Getting more of the breast into his mouth usually solves this problem.

When nipples are difficult for the baby to grasp, we will sometimes use what can be called a "nipple everter." This is made using an ordinary 12 or 20 cc syringe. One takes out the plunger, cuts off the end to which the needle is usually attached, and reinserts the plunger through the newly cut end. The "everter" is then applied to the nipple, and the nipple is drawn out. The advantage this gadget has over a pump to draw out the nipple is that it does not extract the mother's milk at the same time, or only very little milk. If a baby is reluctant to latch on, he is more likely to latch on if he can get milk easily from the breast. If the mother pumps off the first let-down of milk, the baby may be frustrated when he begins to suck because milk isn't instantly available. The effect of the "nipple everter" is temporary. The mother does not have a lot of time to get the baby latched on before the nipple goes back to its usual shape, but still, sometimes the "edge" one gets by using the "nipple everter or extractor" is just enough to get the baby to latch on well. Once the baby is latched on, he will start to pull the nipple out as he suckles. Personally, I do not use this very frequently because it's not necessary, but it is something useful to have in one's stock of helpful devices.

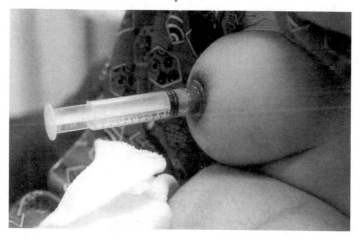

Nipple everter or extractor. Made from a 12 or 20 cc syringe with the end that usually holds the needle cut off and the plunger put in through the resulting hole. This mother has an inverted nipple which comes out very easily with this technique and would and did evert once the baby latched on.

In summary: with regard to nipples and breasts, most mothers have just the right nipples and breasts to breastfeed successfully. It is not right to tell them, as I have heard said not infrequently, that they don't have the right equipment and better not even try.

And a story from Teresa: When my daughter-in-law was pregnant with her first baby, she came over one day and said to me: "I was looking at the pictures of the nursing mothers in the midwife's office and my nipples don't look anything like the ones in the pictures. Am I going to have problems breastfeeding?" Before I could even answer, my son (who was 23 at the time) piped up and said "Oh, I've seen hundreds of women breastfeeding and they have all different sizes and shapes of nipples, and they all work just fine. Don't even worry about it." And of course he was right. Another reason why it's important for women to breastfeed in public!

Breast engorgement

It is worth saying a word about the engorgement that many mothers get on day 3 to 5 after the birth of the baby. I believe strongly that a baby who was "breastfeeding fine" for the first few days and then refuses to take the breast, or starts "latching on" poorly on day 3 to 5, *never* latched on well. Before the breast became engorged, the baby was allowing the breast into his mouth, not really latching on. The baby would suckle briefly and then fall asleep without really getting much milk. This is not latching on. This is pretending, and it's a dangerous bit of business. If the baby continues to do this type of "latching on" after the first few days, the baby can get seriously dehydrated with possibly very serious consequences. Luckily, most babies become agitated and refuse the breast once it's impossible to pretend. They fight, cry, pull at the breast, open wide and try to grab the breast, but cannot. This sort of problem can and should be prevented by getting the baby to latch on well and breastfeed well before the milk normally "comes in" (by day 3 to 5). These early days when the breast is soft and the amount of milk fairly small provide a good situation for the baby to learn to breastfeed effectively. Indeed, if the baby is breastfeeding very well during the first few days, mothers will rarely get engorged to the point of having redness, edema, pain, and most importantly, difficulty getting the baby latched on when the milk comes in. I do think, though, that many of the bad cases of engorgement I see are caused by the IV fluids – it's the mothers who have had an epidural for 24 hours or longer and have been getting fluids all that time who are terribly engorged by day three. It's not having too much milk, so the baby's feeding doesn't make much difference – it's just that they have all this excess fluid. Their ankles are as bad as their breasts.

Nipple shields

Although many lactation consultants use nipple shields to help deal with latching on difficulties with breastfeeding, I find that the kindest thing I can say about them is that they are used too often and too early. I understand that there are, in fact, situations when a nipple shield can be useful, but as with all tools, it can be overused and misused. Many find it a good tool to help latch on premature babies and increase the milk flow to the baby. Perhaps, nipple shield advocates in this context see more premature babies for breastfeeding than I do. But given the evidence of what is possible for getting premature babies to breastfeed-at a much earlier age without the use of nipples shields in such places as Sweden and our own clinic experience, I believe that the routine use of nipple shields is not justified.

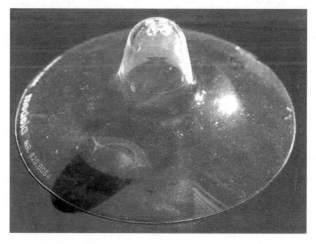

"Modern" nipple shield. It's use should be restricted to those who really have extensive experience helping mothers breastfeed and in my opinion there is no place for its use before the milk supply "comes in" on day 3 or 4.

The worst abuse of the nipple shield, however, is when it is given to mothers whose full term, healthy newborn is only a day or two old but has not yet latched on. To even consider such an intervention before the milk even comes in is a travesty of breastfeeding help. We know that many babies who are not interested in taking the breast or who actively refuse to take the breast will take the breast once the milk supply becomes abundant on day 3, 4, or 5. To suggest the mother use a nipple shield when the baby is only 2 days old is often blocking the possibility of taking advantage of that rapid increase in milk supply only a couple of days later. The use of a nipple shield in this situation is bad practice, nothing less.

I have heard lactation consultants say that if the mother hadn't gotten the baby on to the breast with the nipple shield, she would not have continued. But what happened to counseling? What happened to helping the mother understand that it may still work in a couple of days? Of course, the mother needs to have knowledgeable and skillful followup around 4 or 5 days after birth to take advantage of the increase in milk supply, but what cannot be done on day 2 can certainly be done very often on day 4.

Furthermore, I am convinced that the use of the nipple shield decreases the milk supply. I realize that many people do not agree with me, especially when using the newer "more advanced" models, but I see these mothers and babies at a later stage of breastfeeding than most of those who say the milk supply is not affected. And what I see is that the milk supply has gone down, over time. The problem then is that babies latch on best and most reliably when the mother has a good milk supply. Thus, it is better, I think, that the mother express her milk and give it to the baby than to use a nipple shield. Expressing the milk will maintain the milk supply at a higher level than the nipple shield, and thus the baby is more likely to latch on eventually. If mothers are using a nipple shield, then pumping after each feeding can help to maintain milk production.

When the nipple shield is thought to be necessary, it is imperative that the mother and baby be followed closely by an experienced lactation specialist, both to make sure the baby is getting enough milk and to try to get the baby drinking directly from the breast without the use of the nipple shield. Simply giving the mother a nipple shield on day two and then checking her out of the hospital with no follow-up plans is just not good enough.

Baby problems

Breastfeeding is a two person (sometimes 3 or more) activity, and, of course, the baby may be a major part of the difficulty in getting a good latch or even latching on at all.

Babies may have facial and oral abnormalities that may result in their not being able to latch on well or at all. Amongst these are tongue-tie, cleft lip, and cleft palate. Some lactation specialists discuss "high-domed" palates and "bubble" palates as other causes of poor latches, though I am amazed at how frequently these "special" palates look perfectly normal to me.

Neurological abnormalities in the baby may also result in the baby's not achieving a good latch. Neurological abnormalities may be temporary, as in the baby affected by maternal medication, or longer lasting as in asphyxia or trisomy 21. The baby with trisomy 21, in addition to hypotonia, also has a large tongue (or small mouth depending on how one looks at it). Often, the baby also has cardiac problems which may interfere with his breastfeeding well. Even longer lasting neurological abnormalities may vary with time, usually, as in the case of hypotonia in the baby with trisomy 21, improving as the weeks go by, thus making it easier for the baby to get a good latch at 4 weeks of age, than at 4 days of age.

Cardiac or respiratory problems in the baby, if severe enough, may result in the baby not being able to take the breast well, usually because of tachypnea or congestive heart failure.

Of course, any severe disease may interfere with the baby's latching on well or at all. There is no need to discuss every illness a baby may be born with or develop, but it is important to mention that the possibility of some medical problem other than "the baby just doesn't want to take the breast" should at least be kept in mind when evaluating the baby with breastfeeding difficulties. Since breastfeeding is an essential function in evolutionary and biological terms, if a baby is having difficulties, the possibility of underlying medical problems should always be considered.

Tongue-tie

When the baby has a tight lingual frenulum, it is difficult for the baby to latch on well. Many will call this a short frenulum, but in fact, a short frenulum is not a problem. Rather, it is the long but tight frenulum that causes difficulty, holding the tongue down, and preventing it from doing its job properly; that is, helping to elongate the breast in the baby's mouth and "stripping" the breast of milk.

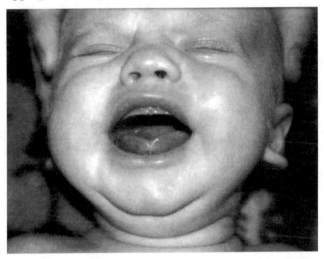

Note baby's heart shaped tongue. The baby's tongue is held down by a tight frenulum.

Why this issue of tongue-tie and breastfeeding has become a battleground between lactation specialists and physicians is something of a mystery. I suspect it is due to the fact that for many years pediatricians cut tongue-ties in babies thinking that tongue-tie interfered with the proper development of speech. Then, when studies showed that tongue-tie, at least the usual mild tongue-tie that is generally seen, does not interfere with speech development, pediatricians were embarrassed by the many unnecessary tongue-tie releases they were doing and rejected tongue-tie as a possible problem altogether. The fact that breastfeeding was never even considered in the rejection of tongue-tie as an issue has been forgotten. In fact, tongue-tie became a non-issue at the very time that breastfeeding initiation in industrialized societies was at its lowest point.

Our experience is that tongue-tie can very much affect the success of breastfeeding because it interferes with the way the baby latches on to the breast. Can babies succeed at gaining well with exclusive breastfeeding if they have a less than perfect latch, whatever the cause? Yes, of course, some will do very well, particularly if the mother has an abundant milk supply and the feedings are not restricted or timed. Can the mother escape without sore nipples even if the baby latches on poorly, for whatever reason? Yes, of course, because a poor latch does not always cause sore nipples. Thus, even if a baby has a tongue-tie which interferes with his latch, breastfeeding can sometimes still go very well. But a tongue-tie still interferes with breastfeeding, and in many cases the resulting problems with milk intake and sore nipples may end up causing early weaning.

If a tongue-tie release involved major surgery, then I would be reluctant to do it. But it is a simple, safe procedure. It takes perhaps two seconds to do the tongue-tie release itself. Explaining to the parents the possible risks – and really a drop or two of blood in about half the cases is all that we see - and how the procedure is done is usually by far the longest part of the whole process.

Although long, complex evaluation tools are available for "measuring" the effect of a tongue-tie on the baby's sucking ability, basically I base my decision on whether it interferes by putting my finger under the tongue, next to the frenulum. If it feels tight, it is tight, and I believe that snipping a tight frenulum will help with any breastfeeding problems.

In theory, the frenulum is bloodless and nerveless and should not cause bleeding or pain for the baby. In practice, often the snip will cause a very small amount of bleeding that will stop as soon as the mother puts the baby to the breast. If one cuts only what is pearly-grey and not what is pink, there should be no problems. However, we do keep a vial of powdered thrombin on hand, in the rare cases when bleeding does not stop. This has occurred twice in 21 years and several hundred tongue-tie releases.

Almost always, babies cry because we hold them down (arms on either side of the baby's face, held tight, so that the baby does not move) but *usually* do not cry more because of the procedure. However, some babies do seem to react to some pain when the frenulum is snipped.

Given the length of time it takes to do the procedure, applying some sort of anesthetic seems to me unnecessary.

Sometimes after the procedure is done, the mother does not see any obvious immediate or rapid improvement. In our clinic, we never simply just cut the frenulum. We also help the mother change the latch; she has almost always been taught to do a symmetric latch (see chapter 2 for how to latch a baby on). We often will give the mothers an ointment for sore nipples and use the Protocol to Increase Breastmilk Intake by the Baby to help the baby get more milk. If the tongue-tie release has been delayed, muscle memory may prevent the baby from changing the way he latches on and/or suckles at the breast.

However, in many cases, the change is immediate. The mother will say that the baby's latch just feels so different and so much better. A baby who was refusing the breast completely, may now latch on. A mother who has had severe pain in the nipples may now be, if not pain free, in much less pain than before - immediately after the procedure! Given the ease with which it can be done, it seems a pity not to include this procedure in the armamentarium of any physician dealing with infants and their mothers.

A couple of emails from nursing mothers:

- *"Though the tongue-tie appeared to be minimal, it was indeed interfering with breastfeeding. I noticed an improvement immediately in terms of contact with my nipple. It took a little time for her to learn she did not need to feed constantly. She is now 7 weeks and everything is much better. Better latch, more efficient feedings, less gas and longer periods of sleep."*

- *"So now, to try to summarize, just 2 weeks ago I finally got to see a pediatrician who clipped her tongue. The latch was totally amazing immediately!!!! Emmaly nurses great now..."*

Cleft lip

In itself, an isolated cleft lip should not cause too many problems with latching on. However, once the alveolar ridge is affected, the problems of latching on become more and more difficult.

When a baby has a cleft lip and difficulty latching on, the problem is often blamed on the cleft lip. However, there are plenty of babies who do not have cleft lips who have difficulties latching on, and babies who have cleft lips may have difficulties for the same reasons (see above). The fact that it is often easy for a baby with a cleft lip to get a good latch suggests that the problem may not be the cleft lip itself.

Some mothers find they can adjust the baby's position on the breast so that the breast "fills in" the cleft lip. Other mothers have used non allergenic tape to close the cleft.

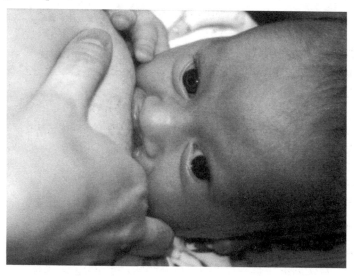

This baby has a cleft lip with extension into the areolar ridge, and guess what, she breastfeeds beautifully. One thing is sure - if one assumes it won't work and the mother does not even try, the baby won't breastfeed.

Cleft palate

A cleft palate is definitely a more difficult problem. In most cases, cleft palates are very obvious at birth. In some cases, though, the cleft involves the soft palate only; the baby's face looks perfectly normal and the problem may be missed. For this reason – as well as many others - all babies should be observed breastfeeding. It is vitally important to evaluate the adequacy of breastfeeding. This should be done with all mothers and babies within a few days of birth at the latest, certainly by the end of the first week. The adequacy of feeding is as important to evaluate as whether or not the baby has a heart murmur, something every baby's doctor would do as part of the routine physical examination. In fact, I believe it is more important since far more babies get sick, some very seriously, and admitted to the hospital because of difficulties with feeding than they do for heart problems. When a baby with a cleft of the soft palate tries to breastfeed, the baby is rarely truly latched on (the breast will usually slip out of the baby's mouth very easily), but with every suck, or virtually every suck, the observer will hear a definite "tsah" or clicking noise. If this is observed, the health professional should make a careful examination the baby's palate as it is very likely the baby has a cleft of the soft palate. In just 2 months at our clinic, we picked up two babies whose cleft of the soft palate was missed, simply by observing a breastfeeding and hearing the "tsah" sound with every suck.

When there is a cleft of the palate, most North American cleft palate teams simply assume that breastfeeding is impossible and that it is not worth even trying to get the baby breastfeeding. I believe this is a pity because, first of all, we do hear of mothers who were able to breastfeed their babies with cleft palates. Perhaps this is a rare occurrence, but it is obvious that if one does not even try, for sure it isn't going to work. I also believe that many mothers feel cheated in not having had the support to give it a try. It is likely that the baby will not latch on, but should not the mother find this out herself after having given it the old college try? I believe she will then accept the inevitable, that the baby just cannot latch on. But when we discourage the mother from even trying, she will always be left with the regret and the suspicion that maybe, just maybe, the baby would have latched on.

This means that attempts to latch on the baby should occur before bottles are given and before the milk "comes in." If necessary the baby can be fed by cup rather than by bottle, preferably with the mother's expressed milk or banked breastmilk. Finger feeding will usually not work with a baby with a significant cleft palate. Neither will a lactation aid, since the baby needs to latch on in order to use the lactation aid. If it doesn't happen, then at least the mother will have tried. This presupposes, of course, that the mother is given expert help, not just the old "give it a go" approach.

In some places obturators are used to fill in the cleft palate for several reasons including, according to those who encourage their use, that repair is easier and speech is often improved when obturators are used. However, though I have no experience with the use of obturators (they are not used at the Hospital for Sick Children in Toronto), their use certainly makes it possible, even likely, that a baby who has one will actually latch on to the breast. Unfortunately, too often breastfeeding is not considered important in a situation when a baby has a major malformation because everyone is so concerned about the malformation. However, helping mothers and babies succeed at breastfeeding is not incompatible with dealing with the malformation. Here is a fertile area for research: how can we best help a baby with a cleft palate (congenital heart disease, cystic fibrosis, meningomyeolcoele, etc., etc.) breastfeed. It was not that long ago that pediatricians were recommending that if the baby was not latching on in the first few days, there was nothing to do except bottle feed. This, after some years of experience, has been shown to be completely untrue. Perhaps, with experience, we will find that some or maybe even many babies with cleft palate can, if helped properly, latch on and breastfeed well. This will never happen if we simply state that it cannot be done.

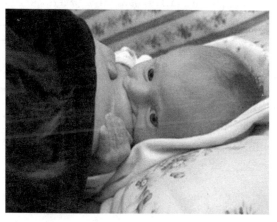

Baby with cleft lip and palate breastfeeding. Maybe a rare case, but if one doesn't try, it will never work.

Nipple confusion

Perhaps this is the place to tackle the contentious issue of nipple confusion. This issue is contentious only because people do not understand breastfeeding. Why it has become yet another battleground of pediatricians against lactation specialists, I have never figured out. There is some emotional baggage hiding in this issue that is obviously driving a lot of the discussion.

Let us look at this logically and calmly. I don't believe that anyone would argue with the statement that some babies prefer a particular artificial nipple, say an Evenflo nipple to a Nuk nipple or vice versa. Or that some babies might prefer a Playtex nipple to an Avent nipple or vice versa, and so on. This is not a radical statement. You don't have to do studies to know that this is true. Just ask any parent who uses bottles. We also don't have to do a double blind randomly assigned study to know that some babies will prefer the mother's right breast to her left or vice versa. When I ask this at conferences at which I speak, about 10%, sometimes many more, of the mothers in the audience will put up their hands to agree that their baby preferred one side to the other. Now, why would a baby prefer one breast to another? There are two likely reasons. One is that the preferred breast produces more milk and the milk flow from that breast is faster. Babies like fast flow, and they will prefer it to slow flow or, and this is important, *slower* flow. Even if the less preferred breast has a good milk supply, the baby will still often prefer the side with a faster flow. A mother who has equal amounts of milk in both breasts (more or less, it's never exactly the same) will not usually have a baby who will prefer one side to the other, even if she has insufficient milk supply. The other reason that a baby will prefer one breast to the other is that the preferred breast is easier to grasp or easier to latch on to. Of course, the fact that the breast is easier to latch on to often results in the breast producing more milk, so the two reasons are related. Are these not the exact same reasons that a baby might prefer a bottle to the breast? Of course. A bottle gives a steady flow of milk, usually quite rapid. The breast can often flow very rapidly, but it is also variable, the flow being fast, particularly during the early part of the feeding, and then slows for a while. Then, the milk flow can increase for a while again, before slowing down, so that milk flow may follow a sort of sinusoidal curve. During the first few days when many babies receive bottles in the hospital (almost always unnecessarily), the milk flow from the breast is hardly ever rapid, but the bottle still is. A hungry baby will figure this one out pretty quickly. "I go to the breast and I don't get very much. Then I get a bottle and I get plenty, even more than I really want. So I'm going with the bottle!" The bonding and closeness are important, but in a baby that is trying to double his birthweight in five months, hunger comes first, especially in the first weeks.

Furthermore, one cannot force a breast into the baby's mouth, or more accurately, one cannot force a baby to latch on to the breast. If one of the mother's breasts is more difficult to grasp, it is usually because the nipple is different (perhaps flatter or inverted, but these reasons only make latching on more difficult, not impossible, see above) from the other side or the breast tissue is different and more difficult to grasp.

One can usually force a bottle into the baby's mouth, even if the baby is reluctant to take it, and the milk flows whether or not the baby sucks. Then the baby must swallow the milk to keep from drowning and that action causes more milk to flow. Indeed, in medical school during our pediatric rotation, we were taught that if a baby was failing to gain weight adequately, we should tip the bottle upside down to see how rapidly the milk flowed. About one drop a second meant the nipple hole was not blocked or flowing too slowly. We were also told to observe a feeding, which is interesting because medical students and pediatric residents are not now taught how to observe a breastfeeding, at least not in most training centres. I'll bet they are still taught to observe a bottle feeding, however.

Taking all the above into consideration, is it really such a leap to assume that a bottle can interfere with breastfeeding, *especially* if the milk supply is low or insufficient?

Thus, it is not the baby who is confused. The baby knows exactly what is going on. The baby who is hungry will prefer the method of feeding that gives him the best reward and in the first few days that is almost always the bottle rather than the breast. Once the milk becomes abundant, however, many babies will accept the breast and latch on reasonably well, but many won't, having gotten used to getting rapid, steady flow from the bottle and the feel of the firm, long nipple in their mouths.

Does nipple confusion or preference mean only that the baby refuses the breast? Not at all, breast refusal is only the most extreme manifestation of nipple confusion. In many cases, it is the final result as well, after other manifestations have made the mother's and baby's breastfeeding experience difficult. In fact, nipple confusion, in my mind, merely means that the baby is not latching on the way he should. The results are often seen in the mother as sore nipples, blocked ducts and mastitis, insufficient milk production secondary to poor nursing or secondary to blocked ducts, and mastitis, which sometimes occurs. In the baby, you see colic, frequent feedings, long feedings even when weight gain is good, poor weight gain and even weight loss, and poor weight gain after an initial good weight gain for 1 to 4 months.

A few emails from nursing mothers:

- *"The last couple of early mornings, Zachary has begun fighting me when I try to get him to nurse. It's like he is saying 'Give me a bottle, it is easier for me and I want it now!' Is this my imagination or is he starting to prefer the bottle over me?"*

- *"In any case, my attempt at breastfeeding is really making me feel like I've failed my six week old son in the breastfeeding feeding department. As you read, I resort to the bottle out of his cries for food. He just won't accept my breast now. I always try to put him on the breast first. Up until 2 weeks ago, I was able to breastfeed him for a while and then I would top it up with the bottle which I knew might lead to trouble, but he was still hungry. Now, he's exclusively bottle fed and I am so disappointed about this.*

One can question here the commonly heard comment "Don't make mothers feel guilty for not breastfeeding." Who actually does feel guilty about not breastfeeding? As these emails (and thousands of others I have received over the years show), it is the woman who wanted to breastfeed but *whom we, as health care professionals have failed*, who feels guilty. Why does no one worry about her feeling guilty?

- *"Hi. I was wondering if you have any advice on coaxing my 5-month-old back to the breast? She receives bottles at daycare and lately is refusing to nurse except for the middle of the night. I'm not ready to wean, but I also can't keep up pumping. As of now she has had no formula."*

- *"While my nipples feel much better (especially a few hours after I apply the gentian violet), they are not totally pain free and they are still red in the centre. As a complicating factor, the gentian violet is irritating my baby's mouth so that she cannot breastfeed, though she will still take a bottle. I should also mention that we have been dealing with thrush since the end of May."*

This one is interesting in that the mother thinks the baby is refusing the breast because the gentian violet is irritating the baby's mouth, yet the baby will take the bottle, even though one would think that the hard latex nipple of the bottle would be more irritating than the soft breast. This is clearly a case of nipple confusion.

- *"I have a one month old son who I was breastfeeding, but due to some weight loss (12%) in his first week my pediatrician suggested I supplement him with formula with a bottle. (The latch wasn't the problem because I had .... a private consultation; I think my milk was just slow at coming in.) Once I did that for about a week, he no longer wanted my breast."*

- *"I have a 10 week old daughter. I have been exclusively breastfeeding her from day 1. I attempted to introduce her to a bottle of expressed breast milk two weeks ago. I would like to be able to have someone else give her the occasional bottle when required. For the past two weeks, I have tried the bottle almost every day and she will take the bottle into her mouth but she will not suck on the nipple. She will play with it."*

This later "problem" is a different one than the breast refusal in that the baby refuses the bottle not the breast. But the point is that some babies do both (though some only pretend to breastfeed and are actually only pacifying at the breast and doing all their feeding from the bottle), some will prefer the bottle, and some prefer the breast. Almost everyone who says there is no such thing as nipple confusion will agree that the baby needs to learn how to take a bottle, otherwise the baby may not take a bottle ever (though I do not see why this is a big problem, especially when women have decent maternity leave and do not have to return to work before 6 months after the birth of the baby, six months being the absolute minimal length of time I would consider "decent" maternity leave – a year is much better).

References

Labor Support

Kennell J, Klaus M, et al. Continuous emotional support during labor in a US hospital. *JAMA*. 1991 May 1;265(17):2197-201.

Scott KD, Klaus DH, Klaus MH. The obstetrical and postpartum benefits of continuous support during childbirth. *J Womens Health Gend Based Med*. 1999 Dec; 8(10): 1257-64.

Labor and Birth Interventions

Lie B, Juul J. Effect of epidural vs general anaesthetic on breastfeeding. *Acta Obstet Gynecol Scand* 1988;67:207-9.

Bond GM, Holloway AM. Anesthesia and breastfeeding—the effect on mother and infant. *Anesthesia and Intensive Care*. 1992;20:426-30.

Mahajan J, Mahajan RP, Singh MM, Anand NK. Anaesthetic technique for elective cesarean section and neurobehavioral status of newborns. *Int J Obstet Anaesth* 1992;2:89-93.

Spigset O. Anaesthetic agents and excretion in breastmilk. *Acta Anaesthesiol Scand* 1994;38:94-103.

Sepkoski CM, Lester BM, Ostheimer GW, Brazelton TB. The effects of maternal epidural anesthesia on neonatal behavior during the first month. *Dev Med Child Neurol* 1992;34:1072-80.

Lieberman E, Lang JM, et al. Epidural analgesia, intrapartum fever and neonatal sepsis evaluation. *Pediatrics* 1997 Mar;99(3):415-9.

Lieberman E, O'donoghue C. Unintended effects of epidural analgesia during labor. *Am J Obstet Gynecol* 2002 May; 186(5 Suppl Nature):531-68.

Lieberman E, Davidson K, et al. Changes in fetal position during labor and their association with epidural analgesia. *Obstet Gynecol* 2005 May; 105(5Pt1): 974-82.

Le Ray C, Carayol M, Jaquemin S, et al. Is epidural analgesia a risk factor for occiput posterior or transverse positions during labor? *Eur J Obstet Gynecol Reprod Biol* 2005 Nov 1; 123(1)22-6.

Klein MC, Gauthier RJ, et al. Relationship of epidural to perineal trauma and morbidity, sexual dysfunction and pelvic floor relaxation. *Am J Obstet Gynecol* 1994 Sep;171(3):591-8.

Supplementation

Grey-Donald K, Kramer MS, Munday S, Leduc DG. Effect of formula supplementation in the hospital on the duration of breastfeeding: a controlled clinical trial. *Pediatrics* 1985;75:514-8. (appalling article)

Schutzman DL, Hervada AR, Branca PA. Effect of water supplementation of fullterm newborns on arrival of milk in the nursing mother. Clinical *Pediatrics* 1986;25:78-80. (bad article)

Glover J, Sandilands M. Supplementation of breastfeeding infants and weight loss in hospital. *J Hum Lact* 1990 Dec;6(4):163-6.

Kurinij Natalie, Shiono PH. Early formula supplementation of breastfeeding. *Pediatrics* 1991;88:745-50.

Nylander G, Lindemann R, Helsing E, Bendvold E. Unsupplemented breastfeeding in the maternity ward: positive long term effects. *Acta Obstet Gynecol Scand* 1991;70:205-9.

Lang S, Lawrence CJ, L'E Orme R. Cup feeding: an alternative method of infant feeding. *Arch Dis Child* 1994;71:365-9.

Fisher C, Inch S. Nipple confusion—who is confused? *J Pediatr* 1996;July:174.

Hill PD, Humenick SS, Brennan ML, Woolley D. Does early supplementation affect long-term breastfeeding? *Clinical Pediatrics* 1997;June:345-50.

Causes of Breastfeeding Difficulties

Hogan M, Westcott C, Griffiths M. Randomized controlled trial of division of tongue-tie in infants with feeding problems. *J Paediatr Child Health* 2005;41:246-50.

Amir LH, James JP, Beatty J. Review of tongue-tie release at a tertiary maternity hospital. *J Paediatr Child Health* 2005;41:243-45.

McBride C. Tongue-tie. (editorial). *J Paediatr Child Health* 2005;41:242.

Ballard JL, Auer CE, Khoury JC. Ankyloglossia: Assessment, incidence and effect of frenuloplasty on the breastfeeding dyad. *Pediatrics* 2002;110 www. pediatrics.org/cgi/content/full/110/5/e63.

Messner AH, et al. Ankyloglossia: incidence and associated feeding difficulties, *Arch Otolaryngol Head Neck Surg.* 2000 Jan;126(1):36-9.

Marino BL, O'Brien P, LoRe H. Oxygen saturations during breast and bottle feedings in infants with congenital heart disease. *J Pediatr Nursing* 1995;10:360-4.

Nowak AJ, Smith WL, Erenberg A. Imaging evaluation of breastfeeding and bottle feeding systems. *J Pediatr* 1995;126:S130-4.

Hörnell A, Hofvander Y, Kylberg E. Solids and formula: association with pattern and duration of breastfeeding. *Pediatrics* 2001;107:e38.

Berg KL. Tongue-tie (ankyloglossia) and breastfeeding: a review. *J Hum Lact* 1990;6:109-12.

Various authors. Tongue tie. *J Hum Lact* 1990;6:122-9.

Danner SC. Breastfeeding the neurologically impaired infant. *NAACOG's Clinical Issues* 1992;3:640-6.

Daly SEJ, Hartmann PE. Infant demand and milk supply. Part 1: infant demand and milk production in lactating women. *J Hum Lact* 1995;11:21-6.

Daly SEJ, Hartmann PE. Infant demand and milk supply. Part 2: the short term control of milk synthesis in lactating women. *J Hum Lact* 1995;11:27-37.

Cox DB, Owens RA, Hartmann PE. Blood and milk prolactin and the rate of milk synthesis in women. *Exp Physiol* 1996;81:1007-20.

Uvnäs-Moberg K, Eriksson M. Breastfeeding: physiological, endocrine and behavioral adaptations caused by oxytocin and local neurogenic activity in the nipple and mammary gland. *Acta Pediatr* 1996;85:525-30.

Engorgement

Nikoderm VC, Danziger D, Gebka N, Gulmezoglu AM, Hofmeyr GJ. Do cabbage leaves prevent breast engorgement? A randomized controlled study. *Birth* 1993;20: 61-4.

McLachlan Z, Milne EJ, Lumley J, Walker BL. Ultrasound treatment for breast engorgement: a randomised double blind trail. *Breastfeeding Review* 1993;May: 316-20.

Hill PD, Humenick SS. The occurrence of breast engorgement. *J Hum Lact* 1994;10:79-86.

Humenick SS, Hill PD, Anderson MA. Breast engorgement: patterns and selected outcomes. *J Hum Lact* 1994;10:87-93.

Evans K, Evans R, Simmer K. Effect of the method of breastfeeding on breast engorgement, mastitis and infantile colic. *Acta Paediatr* 1995;84:849-52.

Nipple Confusion

Mizuno K, Ueda A. Changes in sucking performance from Nonnutritive sucking to Nutritive sucking during breast- and bottle-feeding. *Pediatr Res* 2006;59:728-31.

Gomes CF, Trezza EMC, Murade ECM, Padovani CR. Surface electromyography of facial muscels during natural and artificial feeding of infants. *J Pediatr (Rio J)* 2006;82(2):103-9.

5 Helping Mothers to Learn How to Latch Their Babies

However skilled you may be at helping babies latch on correctly and effectively, ultimately the mother needs to be able to latch her baby on her own. For some mothers, having someone else latch the baby on once or twice will be all they need to "get it" – this experience will show them how the baby is supposed to look, how it is supposed to feel, and the steps to take to get the baby latched well.

Others, though, will find that even though everything worked perfectly while they were in the hospital or at the clinic (and getting step-by-step guidance from you), once they get home, it all falls apart. They can't remember where they were supposed to put their hands or where the baby's body should be in relation to theirs. If the latch isn't good, they don't know how to adjust it.

In societies where breastfeeding is the norm, this is not a problem. Little girls grow up watching mothers breastfeed all around them and by the time they have their own babies they know just how it is supposed to look. They see women with all shapes and sizes of breasts and nipples, and babies of different ages, and they see how the position and latch is adjusted so that it works. In those societies, women rarely, maybe even never, put their babies to the breast with a cross-cradle or football hold, yet the vast majority seems to manage quite well. As a friend from Haiti said when she learned what I did: "I didn't know women could have difficulty with breastfeeding." Of course, many women in North America and Europe will say the same thing, but they say that from lack of experience and thinking if it's natural it's easy, whereas my friend grew up with breastfeeding all around her.

But mothers in our society are at a huge disadvantage. Most of the babies they see are being fed bottles and there is no question that giving a baby a bottle is a very different process than bringing the baby to the breast. The fact that so many health professionals deny the possibility of "nipple confusion" or that so many people do not understand why breastfeeding is more than getting breastmilk into the baby attests to the fact that they don't see how different bottle feeding is. If girls or young women in North America do by chance see a mother breastfeeding, she is likely to be completely covered by a blanket – and even if she isn't, for the girl to actually look at the nursing baby would probably be considered rude.

So when new mothers feel uncertain about how to position their babies at the breast, they naturally fall back to what is familiar – the bottlefed baby. They may also struggle if they have been feeding the baby with a poor latch for several weeks, especially at night or when they are tired. Often at those times they go back to the familiar latch that they were using before they came to you.

Giving mothers a simple handout they can refer to at home is very helpful. Copies of the handouts I use are at the end of Chapter 2, pages 39-43.

Here are some other tips for teaching mothers to latch their babies:

Often it helps to put your hands over the mother's hands, so that she feels exactly what you are doing, how much pressure you are exerting, how you tuck the baby's body in close as you bring the baby to the breast. You might do the actual latching of the baby once by yourself, then again with your hands over the mother's hands, then (perhaps when the baby switches sides) ask the mother to latch the baby while you watch and make suggestions as needed.

Helping the mother understand the reasons why this approach to latching works better is often useful. When she knows the physical principles behind the process, she can more easily adjust the baby's position as needed. You can talk to the mother about how adults eat. In adults, only our bottom jaws are free to move. To get a big mouthful of food, we need to be sure the bottom jaw is well under the food. Get her to try the different positions for feeding. She can see for herself that when we tip our heads forward and then try to open our mouths wide, our tongues naturally tend to go up to the roof of the mouth; but when we tip our heads back and open our mouths, our tongues tend to drop down to the floor of the mouth. This is where you want the tongue to be when baby is at the breast.

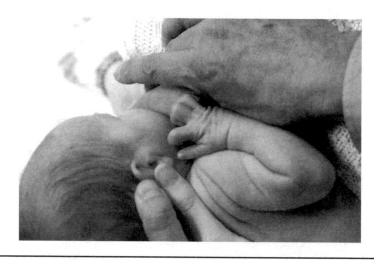

> *Mother has hands placed as previously mentioned. My left hand is on top of hers, guiding her movements so that, one hopes, she will be able to do it herself afterwards. As the baby comes onto the breast, I compress the breast with my right hand, so that the baby gets a gush of milk - I use this compression as the baby comes onto the breast particularly in a baby who is reluctant to take the breast, but it is useful anytime, often resulting in the baby taking the breast with the first attempt, a not inconsiderable advantage if the mother is sore.*

Remind her about what she does when she wants to chug down a drink quickly – tipping her head back and gulping it down. That's what the baby needs to do.

Have the mother take her own finger and feel in her mouth to locate the junction of the hard and soft palate. This shows her how far back in the baby's mouth the nipple needs to go. It also shows her the consequences of not getting it far enough back – the nipple will be pressed against the hard palate and it will hurt! Doing this helps her to realize that even a small adjustment in position and latch can often make a huge difference in how it feels and how much milk the baby gets.

You can let her try to squeeze her breast with her fingers in different places and see how this affects milk flow. If she squeezes close to the base of the nipple, she will likely get no milk at all or only a few drops. If, however, she moves her fingers further back on the breast and squeezes again, she will see the milk spray out. This helps her to see where the baby's gums need to be to compress the breast to get the milk flowing.

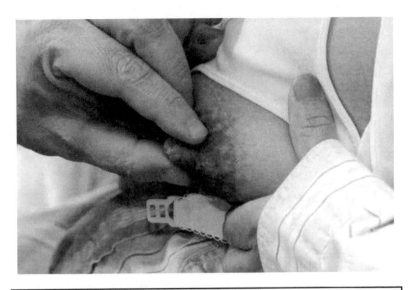

If the baby latches on to the nipple, this is what the baby gets from the breast. Note that I am actually squeezing the mother's nipple fairly firmly.

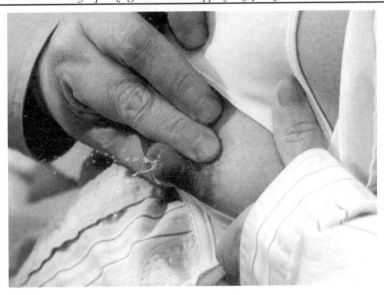

If the baby latches on where he's supposed to, he gets milk. Note that the baby had already "emptied this side." Dr. Jack Newman's Visual Guide to Breastfeeding DVD shows this very dramatically.

These demonstrations and discussions aren't essential, but they give the mother some ways to think about latching that may help her correct any problems that come up when she is at home.

It may also help to warn the mother about some of the more common mistakes or potential problems in latching the baby. Of course, if she has been experiencing difficulties already and if you have watched how she latches the baby normally before beginning to help her, you will already have some points to remind her about. Often it helps to write these down for the mother, giving her a little personalized checklist to go over.

Some common problems:

The mother is pushing the baby's head onto the nipple. This is, unfortunately, often what the mother saw too many nurses doing to her baby every time she went to breastfeed in the hospital, so she naturally feels it is the right way to do it. If her hand is up near the top of the baby's head, she will inevitably be pushing him in nose-first, flexing the baby's neck instead of extending it, so that his chin is away from the breast. Also, most babies will strongly resist having their heads pushed in this way. If it is done firmly enough or often enough, the baby may resist coming to the breast altogether.

The mother has the baby too far over on the side of the breast she intends to feed from. I think this is sometimes an imitation of a bottle feeding position – the baby's head is over by the mother's underarm, or is in the crook of her elbow at her side if the mother is using the cradle hold. In this position, the mother usually ends up pushing his head so that he takes more of the breast above the nipple than below the nipple – just the opposite of what we want. Baby's chin will be tucked into his neck. The ideal position is for the baby to be positioned so the nipple is naturally pointed right at his nose. This means his head is closer to the middle of the mother's body than many women expect.

The angle of the baby's body in relation to the mother's body often needs work. It is less common these days to see babies who are lying flat on their back, although I do sometimes still see this. More often, the mother will have the baby completely tummy-to-tummy. This tends to make it harder to get an asymmetric latch, as the baby is not really able to come on chin-first but tends to come straight on so that he has an equal amount of breast both above and below the nipple. Instead, the baby should be rolled slightly onto his back – not all the way over, but enough that he can look up at his mother's face. If the mother follows the instructions of how to get the "ideal" latch, this slight upward tilt, as well as many of the "angles" we are discussing, happen almost automatically.

This might be a good place to mention the ubiquitous breastfeeding pillow. Many mothers buy these pillows even before their babies are born and have come to think of them as an essential item for breastfeeding. But often the pillows create problems. Many are designed as two semi-circular pieces of fabric stuffed and sewn together, with a seam around each side. This design ends up being like a sagging mattress, thicker in the middle but sloping down towards the mother. Small babies tend to fall into the indentation between the mother and the pillow and often the thicker part of the pillow prevents them from tilting their heads back at all. For mothers with larger breasts, especially if they are also short-waisted, the pillows bring the baby up so high that getting a good latch becomes almost impossible.

Other pillows are designed with a firm block of foam rubber inside, providing a flat surface for the baby to lie on. While this prevents the problem of the baby sliding into the middle, too often mothers end up lying the baby on his back on these pillows, then leaning forward to feed the nipple into baby's mouth. And the problem of having the baby raised up too high is also an issue with this style of pillow.

Not only that, a mother who needs a special breastfeeding pillow to feed her baby is not going to feel very comfortable going out in public. She already has to contend with bringing a diaper bag and other baby paraphernalia, and dragging along a bulky pillow is going to be just too much. And what could be more attention-getting in a restaurant than wrapping yourself in a large pillow before you feed the baby? It just makes breastfeeding seem harder than it really is. I often say (perhaps too often!) you need only a baby and a breast to breastfeed.

If the mother does need some extra support to hold her baby at the breast, she can usually find some pillows or cushions around the house that will work just fine. With her own pillows, she can add or subtract them as needed to get just the right height.

Knowing how to latch a baby on perfectly is only one part of the story. The rest is being able to pass that information on to the mother who will be doing the latching on for the next few years. When she knows why the latch is important and what it should be like, she's better prepared to fine-tune any problems she might run into at home.

6 The Problem of "Not Enough Milk"

Concerns about "not enough milk" are both common and complex. Most people assume that if a breastfed baby is not gaining weight well, then there is something defective about the mother's ability to produce milk. But the reality is much more complicated than that and, in fact, most instances of "not enough milk" are actually a problem of the baby not getting what is available.

The issue of insufficient milk supply is intrinsically interwoven with a whole culture that sees bottle feeding as the norm. Formula company marketing practices have convinced a large portion of our society (including many health professionals who *should* know better) that formula and breastmilk are essentially the same, and that bottle feeding in no way differs from breastfeeding. Birthing practices have affected babies' and mothers' ability to breastfeed. Hospital practices often make breastfeeding difficult, along with the advice and "help" of the staff that are supposed to help mothers. Many health professionals' lack understanding of even the very basics of breastfeeding, including those health professionals who are the ones supposedly "helping" mothers breastfeed (pediatricians, postpartum nurses, midwives, and yes, even lactation consultants). And finally, many health professionals fear lawsuits if they don't follow the "standard of practice," which, with regard to breastfeeding, could hardly be called a standard in any positive sense of the word.

Of course, some health professionals are very knowledgeable about breastfeeding and are able to give mothers good advice and help. Some hospitals have superb practices that encourage breastfeeding and also employ well trained staff to give good help and good advice. But these points of bright light are the exceptions rather than the rule. It is not surprising that many women have difficulty with breastfeeding. Given all the obstacles, it is more surprising that many actually manage to breastfeed successfully *in spite* of the "help" they get. It is not surprising, either, that "not enough milk" is cited in many studies as the most common reason for women weaning.

There are, in fact, *some* women who cannot produce enough milk, in some cases for obvious reasons, but in most, for no known or easily discernable reasons. Some of these reasons will be discussed below. But the most common reason a baby may not grow on breastfeeding alone is not that the mother doesn't have enough milk, but rather that the baby is not getting what is available to him. A baby latched on poorly has more difficulty getting milk from the breast than a baby who is latched on well, and this can be understood (in our bottle feeding society), by imagining a baby bottle feeding with a hole in the bottle nipple that is too small. The baby will take a long time to drink the milk, even though, in theory, there is a limitless amount of milk available to him. By refilling the bottle, in fact, the baby can have available to him multiple times more milk than he could possibly drink at one feeding. As the nipple hole gets smaller and smaller (analogous to a worse and worse latch), the baby gets less and less milk, and may fall asleep with the nipple in his mouth, even though he is still hungry. But if the bottle is taken out of his mouth, he will awaken after a variable period of time (depending on how long and how deeply he was sleeping while sucking), and cry for more food, only to fall asleep yet again while sucking on the nipple that provides little milk flow.

This analogy points out a concept that is a key to understanding breastfeeding: *babies respond to milk flow.* They do not respond to how much milk is in the breast (or the bottle); they care what they get, not the theoretical amount that is available to them. In the extreme case, there is no hole at all in the bottle nipple; the baby eventually becomes dehydrated and, if nothing is done, will die. We see this in "breastfed" babies who become dehydrated in many cases in *spite* of the mother's having plenty of milk. These babies are not breast*feeding*, they are only *pretending* to breastfeed because their breastfeeding is so ineffective that they get no milk, or very little, just as the baby sucking on the bottle with no nipple hole is pretending to feed. I have seen many babies who were admitted to the hospital with severe, even life threatening dehydration who, when the mother was taught the basics of breastfeeding, went on to breastfeed exclusively and to gain weight well, even extraordinarily well.

In most cases, therefore, of "not enough milk" or in more extreme situations, dehydration, the problem can be *prevented* or fixed by fixing the way the baby is latched on to the breast. Yes, it's as simple as all that.

Well, not *always* that simple, as it is not always easy to achieve a good latch. The crucial point is for hospital staff, midwives, and others working with mothers and babies to be able to identify when the latch is good and when it is not good. If there is a problem and they cannot fix the latch themselves, they need to ensure early follow-up for the mother and baby to prevent serious problems. Unfortunately, this is not the situation in most communities.

It is a measure of how little pediatricians know about breastfeeding that during the 1980's and 1990's, many articles came out on dehydration in "breastfed" babies (I wish to emphasize again, that these babies were not breastfed—they weren't feeding at all, just pretending). These babies had hypernatremic dehydration, and when analysis of the mother's milk came back (why did they even do an analysis of the milk?), it was noted that the mothers' milk usually had 5 or more times the amount of sodium than the published amounts of sodium in breastmilk. Conclusion? There was something intrinsically wrong with the breastmilk, it was too salty, and this is what was causing the baby's hypernatremia. This is patently false. The babies were dehydrated because they were not getting milk at all, not high sodium milk, not any milk, and the hypernatremia was due to the fact that the babies were losing pure water (insensible loss) without any replacement (that is, the babies were not getting milk from the breast). If these babies were getting decent amounts of milk, even high salt milk, they would not become dehydrated. Indeed, the amount of sodium in the mothers' milk in these cases was reported to be in the range of the amount of sodium in undiluted cow's milk, which many babies were fed from the very first day of life not that long ago. And babies tolerated it reasonably well, for the most part, *unless* they were put under some stress, such as gastroenteritis. This is a perfect example of how we often measure the wrong things, in this case breastmilk sodium, when we are dealing with breastfeeding.

Why was the sodium so high in the mother's milk? It's simple to explain. "Weaning milk," the milk that the mother produces when the baby is hardly nursing any more, is high in sodium, and this is what was happening to the milk of these mothers—their bodies realized that there was no breastfeeding going on and the breast started to produce "weaning milk." The milk of the breast with mastitis also tends to be high in sodium. The problem is not with the "quality" of milk that the mother produces, nor is the difficulty, in most cases, that the mother is not physically able to produce enough milk. However, there are some situations where physical limitations come into play.

Why some mothers are unable to produce enough milk

We should not be surprised that *some* women are not capable of producing enough milk. After all, some people cannot produce enough insulin and are diabetic. Luckily we can treat deficiencies of insulin, though the treatment, injection of insulin, is far from perfect, and not only because of the need for injections. We just have not been able to duplicate reliably the sensitive mechanism by which the pancreas responds to changes in blood sugar. Luckily for the problem of not enough milk, we have substitutes for breastmilk, but as in the case of treatment for insulin deficiency, the treatment is far from perfect. As a substitute for breastmilk, it would be better if breastmilk banks could be available to provide mothers who were unable to produce enough milk with the better substitute, that is, human milk, rather than highly processed cow's milk or soy beans.

Breast surgery:

Breast surgery is a common cause of a mother's being unable to produce enough milk. In many cases, "esthetic" breast surgery is done without the woman really understanding the implications of what this means to her future ability to nourish her baby and very frequently at an age when she has not really started to even think of babies and breastfeeding.

1. **Breast reduction:** This common surgery frequently affects milk production since it is usually done with a periareolar incision. Any periareolar incision will affect the milk supply, and the more complete the incision, the greater the effect. Our clinic experience is that most women who have had breast reduction cannot produce all the milk the baby needs, but there are definitely

exceptions. In fact, we have had one mother with breast reduction who was able to breastfeed twins exclusively. Even more recently another mother with breast reduction was able to breastfeed twins exclusively. This is certainly an exceptional situation, but I think it is also important that one not assume, *ipso facto*, that the mother's having had breast reduction automatically rules out the possibility of exclusive breastfeeding. Too often, right from birth, mothers are told they must start supplementing their babies because they have had breast reduction. I think this is a bad approach. In the first place, most mothers with breast reduction still produce significant and probably adequate amounts of colostrum, and thus, the babies do not need supplementation in the first few days (*if they are latched on well*). Secondly, how will we ever know if the mother is amongst those mothers who *do* produce enough milk despite their breast reduction if we jump in immediately and start the baby on supplements? Once the mother believes she won't produce enough, it is difficult to stop the supplements. Even in the case of a mother who has not had breast reduction, the psychological effect of being told that the baby is not getting enough can be devastating and makes it difficult to wean the baby from the supplements.

2. **Breast augmentation:** If done by making an incision near the mother's chest wall, then breast augmentation should not cause any difficulty with milk production. Unfortunately, there are too many plastic surgeons who perform augmentation with a periareolar incision, and even though no breast tissue is taken away, these mothers now find themselves in the same situation as the mother who has had breast reduction. This is interesting because the removal of breast tissue in breast reduction surgery is often blamed for the decrease in milk supply, but given these experiences with breast augmentation, clearly other factors are important.

3. **Any periareolar incision:** Whatever the reason for surgery, a periareolar incision may interfere with milk supply. The more complete the incision, the greater the effect. Procedures such as biopsies of breast lumps and drainage of breast abscesses are often done with a periareolar incision. This is really a shame

because these procedures only very rarely require a periareolar incision. I think the surgeons believe the scar is more "attractive," but this is debatable, and in any case, many mothers would refuse this type of incision if they were given the information that it may affect future milk supply.

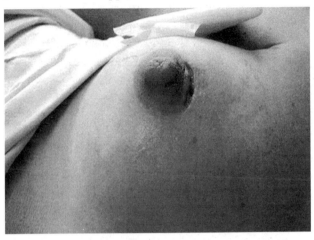

Surgical incision for a breast abscess. So unnecessary and not only prevents return to the breast immediately (because of pain), but also may compromise future breastmilk production.

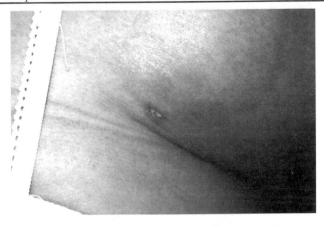

Site of drainage of abscess with a drain placed under ultrasound control. Mother did not interrupt breastfeeding for one minute, even on the affected side. Healing is complete.

Unfortunately, women are rarely given the "straight goods" about any breast surgery they may undergo. Frequently, the surgeon will tell them that the surgery will not affect the breastfeeding at all, though this is clearly untrue. On the other hand, many surgeons will say that the woman will absolutely not be able to breastfeed after having such surgery. This is also untrue. She will be able to breastfeed; she may not be able to breastfeed exclusively. In passing, I should mention that I do not believe that newer techniques of breast reduction, such as not detaching the areola and ducts, result in better milk supplies. This information is being diffused amongst plastic surgeons, who are telling it to their patients, but I do not think we have any good evidence to support it.

Thus, women who are of child bearing age should not have periareolar incisions for any type of surgery if this can be avoided. And it almost always can be. If a nursing mother has had this type of surgery in the past, the adequacy of breastfeeding needs to be evaluated carefully and repeatedly until the situation is clear and further steps can be taken if necessary.

Retained placental fragments:

If a piece of placenta is retained after the birth of the baby, this piece may continue to produce the hormones of pregnancy and inhibit the action of prolactin on the milk producing alveolar cells of the breast. In other words, little milk production will occur. It is not always easy to diagnose the presence of a retained placental fragment. For example, a scan of the uterus is not often helpful because clots and retained tissue sometimes look similar, especially in the presence of infection. Often, the symptoms will be "soft," the new mother complaining only of prolonged vaginal bleeding or vaginal bleeding that had stopped but has restarted. Uterine cramping is more specific, but can be due to other causes. In the presence of such symptoms, a diagnosis of uterine infection is often made and treated with antibiotics. The best way to diagnose retained fragments is still the old-fashioned way, history and physical examination. Poor supply with a history of problems in the third stage of labour, and cramping and bleeding that starts and stops warrants further investigation.

It is hard to know what to make of this. We have certainly seen nursing mothers produce more than enough milk in the presence of a retained placental fragment, probably because it was not functional (that is to say, it was not producing hormones). We have also seen a significant decrease in milk supply that was not corrected with removal of the placental fragment. In such cases, it may be that earlier diagnosis might have made a difference, but this is speculation.

Regardless of how a retained placental fragment is treated, breastfeeding should be maintained and supported. A single dose of methotrexate should not be accompanied by an admonition to interrupt breastfeeding. Long term use of methotrexate should not be considered for a nursing mother, but a single dose or two for treatment of retained placenta, for example, does not require interruption of breastfeeding. Misoprostrol is also sometimes used, and because it has such a very short half-life, it too should not be considered a reason to interrupt breastfeeding. A D&C for removal of the placental fragment should also not result in interruption of breastfeeding, since the medications given during the D&C appear in the milk only in tiny amounts. The mother should resume breastfeeding as soon as she is awake if she's had a general anaesthetic and is feeling up to it.

One mother who had previously exclusively breastfed her twins with no difficulties found she had low milk production after her next baby was born. Eventually, a DNC was done and her milk supply quickly increased.

Endocrinologic syndromes:

a) Sheehan's Syndrome

This syndrome is caused by severe blood loss during labour and birth with resulting shock and, because of the drop in blood pressure, infarction of the pituitary gland. Shock does not always result in Sheehan's syndrome, but if there is a history of severe blood loss during the labor and birth, Sheehan's syndrome should be considered a possibility. The hormones produced by the pituitary gland are of great importance in the maintenance of homeostasis of the body, including the production of milk after the birth of the baby. Sheehan's Syndrome results in partial or total absence of secretion of these hormones. Without prolactin and oxytocin secretion, milk is not produced. However, in the 21st century with modern obstetrics, Sheehan's Syndrome should be a rare event if it ever occurs. It is unlikely that any one of us will be faced with a problem of Sheehan's Syndrome, at least one hopes.

However, I have seen one nursing mother with "not enough milk" who did have partial pituitary insufficiency, probably present before the birth, which was completely atraumatic and not associated with any significant blood loss at all. Her pituitary was intact enough to allow her to get pregnant, but her hormones of lactation were definitely low. Whether this completely explains her problem of insufficient milk production is impossible to say. Suffice it to say that pituitary insufficiency for any reason as a cause of insufficient milk supply is probably extremely uncommon.

One thing we have noticed in our clinic is that women who have been treated in the past with bromocriptine (Parlodel) or cabergoline (Dostinex) for infertility often do not seem to produce enough milk. These drugs inhibit the production of prolactin by the pituitary and are used when the pituitary is overproducing prolactin resulting in infertility (sometimes as the only sign), amenorrhea, and milk production without a previous pregnancy. The treatment often works in the sense that the woman becomes pregnant, but milk production in many such women, who, ironically, were often leaking milk before they got pregnant, is then not up to scratch. It is unfortunate that these drugs seem to have such long lasting effects, at least in some women. I don't think that all women treated with bromocriptine and/or cabergoline have insufficient milk supplies, but I have seen several.

b) Blood loss

The existence of Sheehan's Syndrome has convinced many lactation specialists that any significant blood loss may result in insufficient milk supply. I am not convinced. It is difficult to explain the problem on the basis of pituitary insufficiency, however, if the blood loss was not sufficient to drop the blood pressure significantly and for long enough to damage the pituitary. Perhaps in a mother who would have produced just enough milk, a slight injury to the pituitary, clinically not measurable, could make the difference between "enough milk" and "not enough milk," especially since too often support for breastfeeding in the immediate postpartum period is less than ideal when problems have arisen for the mother (as in the case of significant blood loss) or baby. Perhaps, an explanation may be found in the fact that if the mother loses a significant amount of blood, the fluids are given quite liberally and quite rapidly, and this may result in the baby not latching on well from early on because of edema of the nipple and areola.

c) Polycystic ovarian syndrome (PCOS)

This syndrome seems to be becoming more and more common, or at least more and more commonly diagnosed. It is determined by two criteria: menstrual irregularity and hyperandrogenism. Women with PCOS have oligomenorrhea or amenorrhea, which can cause problems with fertility. The presence of hyperandrogenism can be based on clinical signs such as acne or hirsutism, male pattern baldness, or lab measurements (elevated testosterone or androstiendione). Fifty percent of women with this diagnosis are obese.

Because women with this syndrome have menstrual irregularities, they often have fertility problems. Even in the absence of fertility problems, when women with PCOS have "milk insufficiency," it's tempting to surmise that the PCOS might have a role, and possibly more tempting if fertility has been an issue.

The approach to "milk insufficiency" does not differ in this situation from any other, except that the use of metformin may make a difference. Metformin, a drug used to treat diabetes, is often used in PCOS to help women ovulate and become pregnant. It is also used in these women to treat menstrual irregularities, hirsutism, and obesity. Does it work to increase milk supply? Maybe. Studies are limited, but there have been some encouraging case reports. Metformin acts on a cellular level to increase the activity of the enzyme AMP-activated protein kinase to decrease hepatic glucose production, thus reducing the need for insulin secretion. When insulin decreases, sex hormone binding globulin (SHBG) increases. SHBG, as the name suggests, mops up free sex hormones, including free testosterone. (You also increase SHBG with most types of birth control pills, which is why they work on acne). Additionally, metformin reduces the secretion of insulin-like growth factor, and this hormone seems to cause the ovaries to produce more ovarian androgen.

Why does metformin increase milk production? I don't think anyone really knows, though there are theoretical reasons (see above). Weight loss may be part of the reason, as metformin has been shown in studies to be effective in achieving weight loss on its own or potentiating weight loss achieved by caloric restriction. Most clinicians begin treatment with 500 mg a day taken with a large meal to reduce gastrointestinal side effects. If this is tolerated after one week, add 500 mg the next week, then a further 500 mg to get up to 1500 mg/day. When used for lactation, it may not work straight away. In one study looking at ovulation, some results were seen in the first month of use, so increases in milk production might be seen sooner.

d) Hypothyroidism

Many lactation consultants feel that hypothyroidism is a significant cause of insufficient milk supply. Perhaps. Certainly, it is reasonable to suspect that moderate to severe hypothyroidism could decrease the milk supply, as all bodily functions are decreased with this level of hypothyroidism. But the usual, just slightly low functioning thyroid that we find frequently—does it also cause a decrease in the milk supply? It is hard to know because there is no hard evidence, only anecdotes. Given the general low level of knowledgeable support for breastfeeding and how common slight decreases in thyroid function usually are in women of reproductive age, it is not surprising that many women have coincidental low functioning thyroids at the same time as not having a sufficient milk supply. Is there a cause and effect relationship? Maybe. It makes sense to treat hypothyroidism in nursing mothers. I suspect that treatment of mild hypothyroidism alone will do little if anything to correct breastfeeding problems.

e) Use of feminine hormones by the mother

There is no question that treatment of a nursing mother with estrogens can decrease her milk supply significantly. Birth control pills would be the most common reason for nursing mothers to be taking estrogens. Though the medical literature does not seem to support this statement, our clinic experience, and the experience of many others working with breastfeeding mothers, certainly does.

The problem in many health professionals' understanding seems to be that the decrease in milk supply does not occur in all mothers. In fact, a mother may have a different experience with each baby. Perhaps our clinic experience is skewed in that we would usually not hear from mothers whose milk supply did not go down when they took estrogens. But in some women, there is no question. The chronology is too clear. The mother starts the birth control pill and within a week her previously abundant milk supply has dwindled, sometimes to virtually nothing. No other reasons seem to explain the dramatic drop in what was once an adequate, indeed even an abundant, milk supply in the short space of a week or even less. We have seen this happen in women who nursed, for example, two babies perfectly well while on a birth control pill, only to have their milk supplies disappear with a third baby—same brand and same dose of pill, started after the same time period after birth. Why this one and not the others? We simply don't know the answer.

Many health professionals will acknowledge this effect of the birth control pill, but will suggest that once the mother's milk supply is well established, this is no longer an issue. Wrong. We have seen women start the birth control pill 5 months after birth, with a baby gaining beautifully for 5 months, and all of a sudden, the baby is no longer satisfied at the breast.

Furthermore, I do not believe that the progesterone only pill does not cause a decrease as is claimed by many health professionals. It makes sense that these could be problematic, since progesterone is hormonally active in breast tissue and potentiates the effect of estrogen (even naturally sourced estrogens) in the breast. Perhaps the decrease occurs less commonly, or perhaps we hear of this less because the progesterone only pill is prescribed less often.

It has become the habit of some physicians, particularly in the US, to give new mothers, especially those of low income and/or minority groups, injections of medroxyprogesterone (DepoProvera®) before they are even discharged from the hospital after having had a baby. Dr. Peter Hartmann, working in Australia, has shown that it is the drop in progesterone after the birth of the placenta that sensitizes the milk producing cells of the breast to the effects of prolactin. No drop in progesterone, no milk production. This would explain, at least partially, the failure of adequate milk production associated with some cases of retained placental fragments. But it is of great concern that in order to "assure the mother's compliance with birth control," her caregivers prevent her from developing an adequate supply of milk and essentially force her to supplement or, in too many cases, give up breastfeeding and, incidentally, lose a particularly effective method of conception control, the lactation amenorrhea method.

It is unlikely that the use of topical hormones (as in estrogen-containing skin lotions or vaginal creams) would result in significant absorption of estrogens into the mother's blood, at least not significant enough to affect milk supply, but again, this is based on likelihood rather than on hard data. We have not heard of any significant decrease in the mother's milk supply when using topical estrogens/progesterones. However, we have heard of one case of a decrease in milk supply when the mother had an IUD inserted that released progesterone. This may be coincidental, but it is worth noting.

The issue is that one should avoid the use of the estrogens and progesterones in breastfeeding women. In particular, child spacing methods other than hormonal ones should be the first choice for breastfeeding mothers.

In fact, breastfeeding itself is an excellent method of conception control. Not perfect, but then, neither is the birth control pill perfect. Indeed, tubal ligation and vasectomy are not perfect either, though they are pretty good. **Lactation Amenorrhea Method:** If a nursing mother is breastfeeding exclusively, if she has not yet had a normal period (most physicians would say that any bleeding before 12 weeks postpartum is not a normal period), and the baby is under six months of age, the risk of pregnancy is only slightly greater than with the birth control pill. It's not zero, but it's pretty low, with a 2% failure rate compared to a failure rate of 1% with the birth control pill. If this is too high a risk for the parents, then other methods of conception control may be added - IUD or barrier methods. Rarely is the birth control pill necessary for the breastfeeding mother.

If the mother is on the birth control pill and the milk supply decreases, the mother should immediately stop the birth control pill (not wait until the end of the cycle), and she should start taking domperidone (see more information on domperidone in the section on treatment of "not enough milk"). If the pill has been taken for only a short period of time, stopping the pill and starting domperidone should bring back the supply very quickly, usually within one to three days.

f) Insufficient breast tissue

This diagnosis is made now by lactation consultants when the mother does not seem to produce enough milk and associated with the "insufficient production," the mother has unusually shaped breasts suggesting that the breast tissue is not adequate in volume. The shape of the breast is often described as "tubular" with a relatively wide space between the two breasts. Often the areola is large and there is a groove between the areola and the rest of the breast.

Of course, it is possible that a breast might not have developed in the usual fashion. We see women with one breast that didn't develop as well as the breast on the other side. In fact, it is quite possible that both breasts might have developed incompletely. Whether this has to do with some sort of prenatal hormonal effect, a hormonal effect around puberty in the case of both breasts, or possibly a postnatal injury or infection in the case of one breast is not known. Testicles obviously on one side or both sides can show poor function if they are undescended for a prolonged period of time after birth, though it is also possible that the testicles do not descend properly because they are not normal in the first place.

However, as in the case of breast reduction surgery or any cause of "not enough milk," one should not discourage the mother or begin supplementation unless it is clear that the baby is not getting enough even after going through the Protocol to Increase Breastmilk Intake by the Baby (see page 121). It is rarely clear in the first few days, incidentally. The mother should be helped to get the best latch possible, taught how to know a baby is getting milk, be shown how to use compression to continue the baby breastfeeding, and switch sides when the baby no longer drinks even with compression.

The case of the mother whose breasts are shown in the photos on the next pages is illustrative. She came with her baby when the baby was two days old because she had sore nipples. The nipple soreness was very easy to fix, as you might expect from reading other parts of this book, simply by fixing the latch. The baby did drink a little while at the breast on this visit, but because of the shape of the mother's breasts, I asked her to return in a couple of days. The mother no longer had sore nipples, but the baby, at four days after the birth, still was drinking very little, about the same as during the first visit. The weight had not gone up, but it also had not gone down. So we asked the mother to follow our Protocol and return in a few days. Again, no weight gain, no weight loss, and not very much drinking. I asked the mother to return again in a few days. At 11 days of age, the baby still was at the same weight as at day 2, and even more importantly, I observed no more drinking when the baby was at the breast than a few days before, and this amount was clearly inadequate. I suggested the mother supplement using a lactation aid, but she did so for a couple of days only and then stopped, not wanting to give any formula. For the first month, the baby gained no weight, and the mother and baby did not return for followup. She did maintain contact, however, with our lactation nurse at the clinic, though I was not aware of this. When the baby was four months old, I received a call from the mother who stated that she felt her milk supply was no longer adequate. This was a surprise to me, I thought the milk supply was never adequate. So I suggested the mother return to our clinic with the baby. The photo on the next page shows that the baby was obviously gaining very well. I was truly amazed. In order to reassure myself the baby was actually breastfeeding well, I observed the baby at the breast. She drank beautifully on both breasts, showing that she was indeed getting lots of milk from the breast. It is possible the milk supply was less than it was because decreases in milk supply do occur at 3 or 4 months after birth for reasons to be discussed later. But nevertheless, the baby was getting lots of milk at the breast.

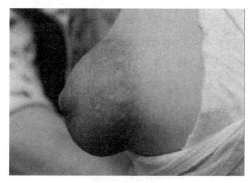

Right breast of a woman whose baby did not gain weight during the first month of life. Note very large areola, notch between areola and breast tissue and seemingly poor amount of breast tissue.

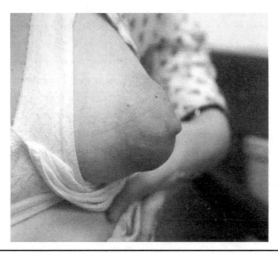

Same woman's left breast. More "breast tissue," but still large areola and notch between areola and breast tissue.

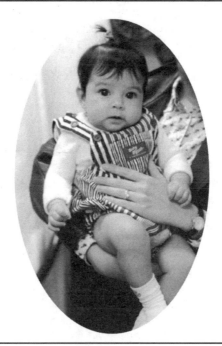

The baby at four months, exclusively breastfeeding and gaining weight very well.

How can this be explained? Especially, how can it be explained in light of a few other women who had breastfeeding experiences similar to this mother, where the weight gain was slow or nonexistent for a few weeks, and then the baby started to gain very well without supplements? Even today, I am not sure what I would suggest in such a case. Suffice it to say that perhaps this notion of "insufficient breast tissue" may be more illusion than real; a special case, perhaps, but not really as big an issue as we generally believe. Perhaps most mothers with "insufficient breast tissue" would have babies follow this same path if we let them. I agree, though, it's difficult to sit back and watch a baby not gain weight for 4 weeks or more. We were able to observe a few such cases only because the mother did not follow our advice to supplement.

Incidentally, one of the speech therapists with whom I once worked came to see me prenatally because, having seen all the mothers with difficulty passing through our clinic, wanted to make sure that she would not have problems. When I examined her breasts, my heart sank. She had the typical breasts of "insufficient breast tissue," even more dramatically than the photos above. And yet she had absolutely no problem, not for a minute, her baby breastfed exclusively and gained weight well.

The most common cause of "not enough milk"

After all is said and done, the major cause of "not enough milk" is the problem of the baby not getting what is available. Why would a baby not get what is available? This might happen for several reasons, often in combination. If only one reason were in play, the baby *might* do very well. This is an extremely important concept which I'm afraid too many people doing research into breastfeeding do not take into account. If the baby has a tongue-tie, it may interfere with breastfeeding, but things may go well anyway because the mother has a lot of milk. If the mother has an adequate but not abundant milk supply, breastfeeding might still go reasonably well, but with more difficulty. If the baby also is getting bottles, for example, the whole system may collapse and the baby may fail to thrive.

The better the latch, the more milk the baby will get from the breast. This is especially true when the milk supply is less abundant. When the milk supply is abundant or even "overabundant," the baby may have a very poor latch and still get plenty, but he will have to depend on the milk ejection reflex (or letdown reflex) to get the milk. As most mothers can have several milk ejection reflexes during each feeding, the baby may gain weight well, even with a poor latch. But the baby may also spend long periods on the breast, the baby may return frequently to the breast, or both. This, of course, is one reason that mothers/health professionals may believe there is insufficient milk. Because the baby is frequently on the breast for long periods of time, mothers are often encouraged to supplement. With supplementation, the baby spends less time on the breast and feeds less frequently, giving us "proof" that there wasn't enough milk. But the reality is that there was plenty of milk – the baby just wasn't able to get the milk effectively.

Or, the mother might hear the other commonly given bit of advice: "Feed the baby only every 3 or 4 hours, so that the milk builds up in the breast and the baby drinks better." This person at least understands that babies respond to milk flow, and a fuller breast often gives faster flow, at least at the beginning. As with many bits of advice given to nursing mothers, this one will occasionally work, so many are convinced that supplementation is necessary or that waiting between feedings is a good idea. However, does it make sense to make a baby wait, allow a baby to cry, or give the baby a pacifier until the allotted time has passed? This is completely contrary to nature - a need requires a response. One eats when one is hungry, the pancreas produces insulin in response to higher blood sugars, the stomach produces hormones and acid in response to food in the stomach, and so on. Though, for some obscure reason, we look at "psychological need" differently (don't spoil the baby). The need for tenderness, love, and being held needs an appropriate response, too. So even if waiting to feed may on occasion work, it is not the right approach because the baby's needs are not met, and there are better ways to do this.

Because mothers often receive poor information, babies often do not nurse well at the breast. Poor nursing results in the breast being less than adequately "drained." While the breast is never actually "empty" when insufficient milk is removed, the message the breasts receive is "make less milk." This results in a decrease in the milk supply, which results in poor nursing, and further decreases in milk supply. Too often supplementation by bottle is added into the mix, and the milk supply decreases even more as the baby takes less from the breast, not least because the bottle nipple results in his not latching on to the breast even as well as before. The vicious circle is in place. However, too often, even when the supplementation is given by alternative methods, the supplementation was not necessary in the first place. In this case where the supplement is not necessary, even if given by lactation aid, it is inappropriate.

Just because the milk supply was adequate or even more than adequate at the beginning, does not mean that it is simple and easy to get the milk supply back to adequate. How easy it is to bring back the milk probably depends on the initial milk supply and how long poor nursing has been the rule for this nursing couple.

Protocol for "not enough milk"

Over the years, our experience with thousands of nursing mothers has led to the development of a Protocol for "not enough milk." If you don't understand the use of the quotes around "not enough milk," please re-read the previous information. The fact is that the most common cause of "not enough milk" is not the mother's physical incapacity to produce sufficient amounts of milk, but rather that the baby is not getting what is available to him. (Have I repeated this too often yet?) However, it is certainly true that if the baby has not been feeding well (and therefore not taking much milk), the mother's milk supply may now actually have decreased secondary to the poor feeding.

The following Protocol works whatever the age of the baby: 1 day, 3 weeks, 3 months, or 30 months. The principles are the same. The principles are the same for twins or triplets, too, though the logistics may be different. The approach also works for premature babies, babies with Trisomy 21, and babies with cardiac disease, etc.

Protocol to Increase Breastmilk Intake by the Baby:

Step 1: Get the best latch possible

It has been mentioned multiple times throughout this chapter and other chapters, since this book is about latch, how important the latch is not only to prevent sore nipples, but also to help the baby get more milk.

Of course, as mentioned previously, if the mother has an abundant milk supply, the baby does not have to latch on perfectly in order to get enough milk. Often the milk supply is so abundant that the baby hardly has to latch on at all, the milk just pours into his mouth. It is for this reason that women have always been able to breastfeed throughout history and around the world without resorting to books or breastfeeding clinics - most women produce more than enough milk, and if breastfeeding is not restricted (by so-called guidelines such as 15 minutes on each side, no more frequently than every two hours, etc.), the vast majority of babies will do just fine breastfeeding exclusively.

Here is an email (pasted here exactly as it was sent to me) I received on March 31, 2006. It is obvious that even at this date, women are getting the numbers treatment. This mother obviously seems to have a sense that she was told nonsense. And she is right. This mother gave birth in Toronto, where I have worked for 22 years to try to get rid of such silliness. But the allure of the numbers is too strong to resist, even if nonsense.

> *"I have a son now who is 3 days old. I was told in the hospital that I should spend 15 minutes on each breast with him. Do I have to do this? I wasn't sure. What if he feeds 20 minutes contentedly on 1 side and doesn't want any more milk? Should I pump out the other side? I know my milk is coming in because I can feel the let down and I know that he's drinking well. I see the deep swallow."*

And the answer is no, she shouldn't pump the other side unless she becomes uncomfortably full and the baby doesn't want any more (the baby is better than any pump when he latches on well).

A better latch also prevents and treats sore nipples and allows the mother to put in the effort that may be necessary to get her baby gaining adequately. It is difficult indeed to "feed the baby on demand" when breastfeeding hurts. So, not only does a good latch help prevent and treat sore nipples, but because the baby gets milk more efficiently with a better latch, the baby feeds less frequently or for shorter periods of time. In fact, some mothers may be able to feed the baby on just one breast at a feeding. However, there should not be a rule about this. The mother should "finish" one breast, and if the baby wants more, the baby should be offered the other side. How does the mother know the baby has finished one side? By the length of time the baby is on the breast? No! By the fact that the baby is falling asleep at the breast? No! By the fact that the baby is not getting any more milk at the breast, even with compression? Yes! Compression is discussed below but is not necessary for all mothers and all situations. We use it in the clinic because we only see mothers who are having problems, and compression is helpful for almost all breastfeeding problems, including "not enough milk," sore nipples, colic, and combinations of the preceding. If all is going well without it, of course, there is no need to use this technique. How to distinguish between a baby getting milk from the breast rather than simply sucking at the breast without getting milk is described below as well. This can be seen on video at www.breastfeedingonline.com, www.gentlemothering.ca, www.thebirthden.com/Newman.html, or in our instructional DVD for breastfeeding. How to achieve a good latch is discussed in chapter 2.

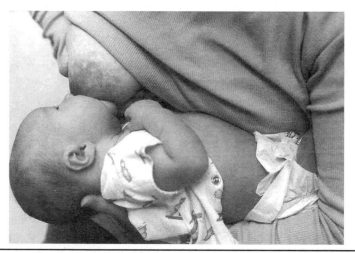

Good cross cradle hold. Good latch. As an exercise, point out the features of the good position and good latch.

This brings us, however, to another example of how a "little knowledge is a dangerous thing." Many breastfeeding specialists have adopted this notion of "if it hurts the latch is no good" with a vengeance. Their solution, which may be worse than the problem, becomes: "Take the baby off the breast and latch him on again. Still hurts? Then the latch is not good. Take him off and latch him on again..." And again and again. The result? Instead of 1 painful latch, the mother has 4 or 7 or even more. This means 4, 7, or even more times as much damage to the nipple, 4, 7, or more times as much pain, a frustrated mother and baby, and often, so much pain so early on in breastfeeding that many mothers will stop or adopt the approach of taking the baby off the breast to give the "nipples a rest." The "nipple holiday" approach to sore nipples is a losing approach in most cases.

There is no guarantee that 3, 4, or even more days of not breastfeeding and giving the baby milk from a bottle in order to give the nipples a rest will improve the baby's latch in any way. Indeed, it is probable that the latch will be as bad as it ever was, perhaps even worse, since the baby has now received bottles for several days, using a very different sucking technique. Indeed, some babies will have started to prefer the bottle and then refuse the breast altogether. Our experience confirms that many mothers may have less pain after several days of no breastfeeding, but often enough, once the baby starts going back to the breast, the pain often returns.

Step 2: The mother needs to know how to know a baby is getting milk from the breast

This knowledge is crucial (see video clips at www.breastfeedingonline. com or www.gentlemothering.ca, or see our instructional DVD, *Dr Jack Newman's Visual Guide to Breastfeeding*) and is sorely lacking in most teaching about breastfeeding. It seems that too often everyone simply assumes that if the baby is sucking at the breast, then the baby must be getting milk. How else can one explain the inane notion that a baby gets 90% of the milk in the first 10 minutes (still current in some circles incidentally)? Simple observation will often show that the baby is getting significant amounts of milk long after 10 minutes are up. How else can one explain the bizarre approach to dealing with "not enough milk" that suggests to a mother that the baby should nurse from one side only, so the baby gets the high fat milk. Here's a secret. If the baby is not getting any milk, the baby is not getting high fat milk. Thus, the mother should give the baby the other side. Two times as much low fat milk, in the context of a baby not gaining well, is better than one time as much low fat milk. If this seems obvious, it is a measure of how in a desirable but misguided effort to make breastfeeding scientifically based, we throw out common sense (with the baby?). Incidentally, there is no such thing as no-fat breastmilk, even the first drops contain some fat.

Once the mother knows how to know if a baby is getting milk, she also knows how to know when the baby is not getting milk, and she can then cut through much of the strange teaching that is frequently given about breastfeeding. Examples abound. For example, mothers are frequently taught to feed the baby 20 minutes on each side. This is a fascinating idea. Since when does timing have anything to do with eating? You can sit down to most meals and finish eating in 20 minutes. But you can also sit down to the same meal and take 60 minutes. Does taking 60 minutes mean that you ate more food? Of course not. The same for breastfeeding. A baby who feeds well for 20 minutes on one side may not take the other side. A baby who spends most of the time nibbling at the breast may spend 20 hours at the breast and still not have had enough. It's not how long, it's how well a baby is breastfeeding that matters.

Many hospitals have policies that require supplementation if the baby loses more than 10% of their birth weight (7% is sometimes used, occasionally 5%). This too makes no sense if one looks at how the baby is breastfeeding rather than the weight. In the first place, scales can be wrong. If the baby is weighed on one scale and then the following weight is on another scale, this tells us nothing. Different scales frequently give very different results. The difference between 9% weight loss and 10% weight loss in a 3 kg baby is only 30 g. Eighty grams difference between different scales is not rare, and 30 g difference is quite common.

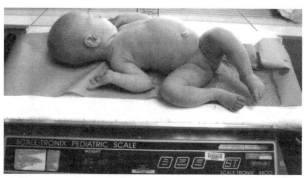

Baby weighed on just verified accurate scale. Note weight 3.51 kg (about 7 lb 12 oz).

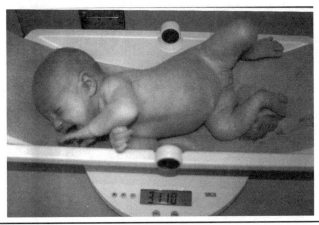

Same baby, less than 5 minutes later, weighed on another, relatively new (3 month old) scale. Note weight 3.11 kg (6 lb 14 oz, rounding up). This scale is used by the pediatric outpatient department of a large Toronto hospital. If a baby is referred for dehydration, the baby is weighed on this scale. How often are scales wrong? Don't ask. How often are mistakes in weighing made? Much more often than is thought. How often are the weights recorded incorrectly? Often.

If instead of looking at the scale, we watch the baby at the breast, we can see whether the baby is actually getting milk. The pause in the baby's chin can be seen, even during the first day, if you know what to look for. If the baby is drinking, even a little, this is of great significance and we and the mother should be reassured. There is no good data that tells us that it is fine to lose 6.9% but that 7% is too much. The difference between 6.9% and 7% in a 3 kg baby is 3 grams, within the range of error of most scales. This should not be a license to start dropping the allowable % weight loss lower and lower, however, as has happened in some maternities. "The baby lost *almost* 7%, so we had better supplement." "6.5% is almost 7%, maybe we should lower the allowable weight loss to 6%, just to be sure." How does one deal with this issue? Fix the breastfeeding! Follow the Protocol to Increase Breastmilk Intake by the Baby!

Here is a recent example, yet again from Toronto (how embarrassing). We saw a 2 week old baby at the breastfeeding clinic on March 27, 2006, because the mother wanted to get the baby off the nipple shield she was using (started when the baby was three days old, something I find perfectly appalling and according to what the mother was saying, it was not even clear why the nipple shield was started). The parents stated that the baby weighed 4.15 kg (9 lb 2 oz) in the delivery suite. Thirty minutes later, the baby was re-weighed on another scale and had lost 180 g (6 oz). In spite of this confusion, the next day (the baby was barely 24 hours old), the baby was re-weighed, the parents were told that the baby had lost 8% of its birth weight, and the mother had to supplement. The parents refused, quite rightly noting that nobody knew what the baby's birth weight actually was. Did anyone watch the mother breastfeed? No. Are we in the Twilight Zone of breastfeeding here? Yes! Incidentally, in spite of the mother using a nipple shield, the mother had a lot of milk and the baby was growing well (and drinking well at the breast in spite of the nipple shield). Does it make sense that a mother with this large supply would not have enough colostrum?

Step 3: Use compression to "finish" the first side and then offer the other

Once the mother knows when the baby is getting milk, she will also know when the baby is *not* getting milk. Hoping I am not repeating this too often, I would like to remind the reader that a baby is not getting milk from the breast simply because he is latched on and making sucking motions.

Thus, when the flow of milk starts to slow and the baby does more and more nibbling at the breast and less and less drinking, many babies, especially in the first few weeks, of life will tend to fall asleep at the breast. This does not mean that they are full, necessarily. They might be, but they may only be responding to the decrease in milk flow. Thus, many new mothers are surprised that when they take the sleeping baby off the breast, the baby starts to cry with hunger again. "But, he's already been nursing for 30 minutes. He *must* be full." Not necessarily. Again, the baby is not necessarily getting milk just because he's sucking, even though he's been on the breast for 30 minutes. He might have actually only been drinking for 5 minutes (don't count the minutes).

As they get older (say older than 4 or 5 weeks), many babies instead of falling asleep at the breast when the flow of milk is slow may actually pull at the breast, especially if they are quite hungry. This is of importance because many mothers interpret this as meaning that the milk is drying up, but in fact, what has changed is the baby's behaviour, not the milk supply, at least not usually. It is also important because I think it explains many cases of why some babies do not gain weight after 2 or 3 months of exclusive breastfeeding even though they gained very well for the first 2 or 3 months (see chapter 10, Slow Weight Gain after Initial Adequate gain).

Babies pull or cry at the breast and get angry for several reasons:

1. The flow is too slow.

2. The flow is too rapid.

3. The baby is full, but wants to continue to suck. This often occurs when the mother has an abundant supply, and the baby nurses so quickly that his sucking needs are not met.

4. It is possibly due to a reaction to something in the milk.

5. The baby is having a nursing strike.

6. Reflux is a possibility here, but this is a "diagnosis" which is made too often.

7. A combination of 1 and 2 (too fast early in the feeding, too slow later).

You can decide which of the first three is causing the baby to pull at the breast by watching the baby drink at the breast. If the baby is nibbling, it is likely 2. "I want more milk faster." If the baby is drinking, it is probably because the flow is too rapid for the baby to handle (this usually occurs early in the feeding), or a variation of the baby is full, got full very quickly, and wants to continue to suck but does not want more milk. Number 3 usually occurs several minutes into the feeding when the baby was drinking very well. Often the baby, after the initial rapid drinking, is content when nibbling and not getting much milk, but if the milk flow begins again, the baby will start to get upset.

The problem of too slow flow is improved by improving the baby's latch, using compression, and possibly using other tricks to increase flow (herbs, medication). Domperidone could be helpful in this situation, but should be used *in conjunction with* the Protocol not as a "magic bullet."

The problem of too rapid flow is improved by improving the latch and letting time do its work. Feeding on one side at each feeding may help. Eventually, by 2 to 3 months at the most, the baby will learn to manage the flow.

The problem of the baby being full can be improved by "finishing" one side before offering the other and trying two or even more feedings on one side. For example, all feedings within a period of say four hours are given on the left breast. Then for the next four hours, all feedings are given on the right breast. The mother needs to be sure that the baby is getting enough milk this way and is not hungry. If the baby seems hungry and is no longer drinking at the first breast even with compression, she should offer the other breast.

The problem of reflux can be treated with medication if the above approach to too rapid flow cannot be fixed. (It's better for the baby to get reflux medication than the medication called infant formula.)

So, when the flow slows, instead of allowing the baby to "nibble himself to sleep," the mother starts using compression to increase the flow of milk again. This technique works particularly well during the first few days when the milk supply is certainly adequate, but not abundant. The mother starts compression when the baby sucks, but *does not actually drink*. A frequent error is made when mothers compress when the baby is not making any sucking motions at all. This will get the baby to start sucking because some flow of milk into the baby's mouth will encourage him to suck. But if the mother uses compression when the baby is already sucking, then mother and baby are working together.

We find that compression works best when the mother gets a good handful of breast and again, *as the baby sucks but does not drink* (no pauses in the chin), the mother compresses the breast, using her thumb and the flat of her hand (see photo page 138). If this works, the baby will start to drink again. The mother continues the compression until the baby stops sucking or the compression does not result in drinking. She then releases the pressure or the compression. Usually the baby will stop sucking if he hasn't already. The baby will restart sucking when he tastes some milk and the mother repeats the process. A video clip of this can be seen at the previously mentioned websites as well as in the DVD *Dr.*

Jack Newman's Visual Guide to Breastfeeding.

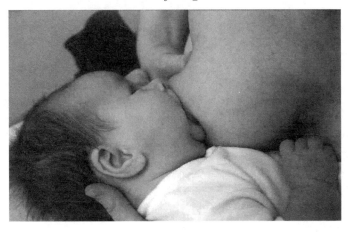

The mother squeezes the breast with her hand as the baby sucks, but does not drink. There is no need to push towards the baby as this may cause the mother pain or injure the skin.

How long should the mother continue the compression on the first side? Until it does not work any more. That is, until the baby does not drink even with compression. It is not an easy question to answer because mothers can have several milk ejection reflexes at each feeding. It is not rare for a baby not to drink much for several minutes and then start drinking a lot all of a sudden as the mother's milk lets down. I am convinced that compression not only *simulates* a milk ejection reflex (external rather than internal milk ejection reflex), but can actually stimulate one as well. It is not rare to see a mother start a compression and before she really has compressed the breast, the milk starts to flow rapidly as confirmed by the baby's drinking and drinking. However, if the baby is getting sleepy or, on the contrary, starts pulling at the breast and compression is not getting more milk into the baby, then changing sides makes sense. There is no reason to say 20 minutes on the breast or 30 minutes on the breast. When the baby no longer drinks reasonable amounts even with compression, switch sides.

When the baby is not gaining well, this is not a reason to suggest one breast at a feeding. I have mentioned this already, but it needs emphasizing. The mother should "finish" the first side and then offer the other side. In fact, this should be an approach to all breastfeeding situations, even when everything is just fine. How does the mother know the side is "finished"? The baby doesn't drink any more even with compression. However, if all is well, there is no need for the mother to use compression. Waiting until the baby is fast asleep may result in the baby not seeming to be interested in the other side. Again, common sense needs to rule. Most of the time, when a baby doesn't gain, it's because he is not getting enough milk (of course, there are other reasons, including illness, but this issue cannot be dealt with here). Thus it makes sense that the baby would want and would need at least both breasts. And on the second breast, compression will help, too. In fact, there is no reason (except nipple soreness) that a baby cannot go back to the first side to drink again. It is frequently observed that a baby who was no longer drinking on the first side, goes to the second, and returns to the first and drinks a lot of milk again.

Often, that is all that is necessary, and babies will start to gain well. In most cases supplementation will not be necessary or desirable. If the baby drinks very well, he will probably gain well. If the baby drinks not at all, supplementation will likely be necessary. But what if the baby falls in between—the baby drinks some, but not a lot and spends considerable time just nibbling? Then he will be all right for a day or two, there is no need to rush into supplementation. Follow the above Protocol and most babies will, in fact, do fine. Close followup is necessary, however. It is worth using herbs to help increase the milk flow.

Step 4: Herbs do seem to help

We usually suggest the mother start with 3 capsules each, three times a day, of blessed thistle (*Cnicus benedictus*) and fenugreek (*Trigonella foenum-gracus*).

For many years now, we have used blessed thistle and fenugreek to help mothers with "not enough milk." There is a bit of research to show that fenugreek increases milk supply, but we do not have studies on these two herbs taken together. However, our observations suggest that they are effective. Perhaps this is a placebo effect, but if it is, does it really matter? Many years ago, a wise breastfeeding advocate stated that "breastfeeding is a confidence trick." Well, not completely, but there is no question that confidence and support are very important, and if these herbs do nothing but give confidence, it's not such a bad thing, is it? But in fact, I think they do work, at least for some mothers. No drug, incidentally, works for everyone. When drug trials are published and 90% of patients respond to a drug, this is considered a very good response. But it still means 10% do not.

We find that blessed thistle and fenugreek work best in the first few days or weeks (generally 2 to 4 weeks) after the baby's birth. But they do seem to work well with some mothers who had a late onset decrease in their milk supplies for the reasons mentioned in chapter 10.

Other herbs, which others have used and the value of which is not particularly well documented either, are: goat's rue, marshmallow leaf, raspberry leaf, fennel, and alfalfa. We tend to use only the fenugreek and blessed thistle because we have experience with them. We cannot ask mothers to buy all the above herbs for monetary reasons and because they are not always easy to find. Furthermore, even though these drugs are natural source drugs, they are still drugs if they have an effect on the body. And natural source drugs can be as toxic as any other sort of drug. The more different drugs one takes, the more likely it will be that one will get a serious reaction. And we should not forget the practical issue of taking several drugs. Fenugreek capsules, for example, are very big pills to swallow, a not inconsiderable problem for many mothers.

There are rumours that fenugreek can cause lowering of the blood sugar and increase the severity of asthma. Furthermore, some people say that women with peanut allergy should not take fenugreek. I have never seen evidence for any of this and, in our experience, reactions of any sort are very uncommon with fenugreek. Some women definitely get abdominal cramps with fenugreek, but this problem settles after a few days even if the mother continues the fenugreek. Some women have gotten rashes while on fenugreek without evidence that it was, in fact, the fenugreek that caused the rash.

Side effects due to blessed thistle seem to be extremely rare, and often side effects noted by the mother may not be due to the blessed thistle. Blessed thistle is different from milk thistle, an herb used for "cleansing of the liver." Some people claim that it too increases milk supply, but we have no experience with it.

Fenugreek has a very distinct odor, which the mother will be able to detect emanating from her skin. In fact, we use this fact to determine if the mother is taking enough fenugreek—if the mother's skin does not smell of fenugreek, she is not taking enough. Herbs sold in North America are not standardized and dosage of active ingredients (if there are any) may not be the same regardless of how much fenugreek or blessed thistle is said to be in the capsule. A capsule of 705 mg (why the "5," I'm not sure), may actually be less potent than a capsule of 505 mg with regard to its effect on milk supply.

How long a mother takes the herbs must be determined by the clinical situation, not some arbitrary time limit. If, after following this Protocol and taking the herbs, things are going well (the baby drinks well, the baby is gaining well on breastfeeding alone), the mother can start weaning herself from the herbs. We don't know if gradual reduction of the dose prevents a drop in the milk supply, but, generally, it is prudent to stop the herbs slowly rather than suddenly. Weaning off the herbs over a period of a week or two seems reasonable.

One more practical issue: herbs, not being prescription drugs, are not covered by drug plans. Domperidone (see page 137) usually is. For parents with limited financial resources, the cost of the herbs, though not excessive, can nevertheless be a real burden. In such situations, it may be better to use domperidone.

The following is a summary of the information on fenugreek and blessed thistle.

- Fenugreek and blessed thistle seem to work better if the mother takes both, not just one or the other.

- Fenugreek and blessed thistle work quickly. If they do work, the mother will usually notice a difference within 3 to 4 days of start to take them. If not, they probably won't work.

- Fenugreek is often sold as a combination with thyme. It is better to use fenugreek without thyme.

- Herbal remedies are not standardized, so though the bottle of fenugreek, may say that it contains 405, 505, 605 or 705 mg/capsule. We do not really know how much of the active ingredient you are taking. Fenugreek has a distinct smell. If the mother or others cannot smell it on her skin, the mother is not taking enough, even if she is taking three capsules three times a day.

- Fenugreek and blessed thistle seem to work better in the first few weeks than later on. In fact, they tend to work best in the first week. Domperidone works better after the first few weeks.

- Mothers can take fenugreek and blessed thistle together with domperidone if both seem to be helping. If the mother takes the herbs and domperidone, it is probably better she take the domperidone at the same time as the herbs, for example, 3 tablets three times a day.

- Fenugreek does not cause low blood sugar. Where this rumor came from is unknown.

In our experience, the above four steps will work in the majority of mothers suffering from the problem of "not enough milk." Of course, as mentioned earlier, some mothers are incapable of producing enough milk for several reasons (and some, for no reason that we can discern), but these steps will usually allow the baby to get more milk than what the baby was getting beforehand. Thus, any supplementation requirements will probably be reduced.

Other steps the mother can take are the following. Most mothers seem to have less milk in the evenings. Whether there is a physiological basis for this or it is due to fatigue is not really known. There are data to suggest that the fat content of milk is less in the evenings, and this may explain babies' wanting to be at the breast frequently or for long periods of time, or both, in the evening. This can be very upsetting to parents, who have too often been led to believe that babies should not feed more often than every "x" hours or no longer than "y" minutes on each side. But, if there is a question of "insufficient milk," these evening feedings can destroy the parents' confidence and lead to unnecessary supplementation. This is a good time for the mother to lie down with the baby, side by side, and let the baby nurse for as long as he wants. The mother may even fall asleep while the baby nurses and why not? If she gets more sleep, this will help her milk supply. Furthermore, if the baby sucks for 3 hours in the evening and the mother is sleeping, she won't know how long the baby was at the breast. If the mother is not yet able to feed lying down (it is not that complicated and the father can be invaluable in helping the mother get the baby latched on in this position), then renting and watching long movies (e.g. *The Ten Commandments*, 3 hours 40 minutes) can be a way not to worry about the length of time the baby is at the breast.

Should the mother express or pump her milk to augment the milk supply? In theory, this is a good idea. In practice, it does not always work out that way, and too many mothers have quit breastfeeding altogether because they could not keep up the pumping schedule advised by many lactation consultants. To tell the truth, I am not keen on pumping in this situation for the following reasons (there are other very valid reasons, of course, to express milk, such as for a baby who is too premature to breastfeed or when the baby is refusing the breast):

1. Pumping is expensive (to rent or buy the machine).

2. Pumping is tiring and time consuming.

3. Pumping diminishes the mother's enjoyment of breastfeeding.

This is very important. Mothers have frequently expressed to me the frustration of doing nothing but feeding. "I feed him 30 minutes on each side (why 30 minutes?), then I express my milk for 30-45 minutes, and by the time I've finished, the baby wants to nurse again."

4. Pumping, if not done properly, can cause sore nipples.

5. In spite of everything we tell mothers about not being able to tell how much you are producing or can produce by the amount you can pump, mothers look at the volume of milk they pump and get discouraged.

6. Compression (see page 127 of the Protocol to Increase Breastmilk Intake by the Baby) is like pumping, but instead of pumping into a bottle, the mother expresses into the baby. It works even better, in my opinion.

What if the above does not work and the baby still does not gain well enough?

The first question is what is "not gaining enough"? It is important to remember why we follow babies' weights. It is not just to make a pretty graph. It is not because the baby needs to keep on his percentile, come hell or high water. The reason for a growth chart is to help us pick up on medical problems in the baby. If a baby was on the 25th percentile for a few weeks or months and then drops to the 3rd percentile, this, *in itself*, is not an indication for supplementation. Supplementation will not do anything for the baby's coarctation of the aorta, for example, or for the baby's urinary tract infection. Though most of the time the issue is due to feeding problems, it is not a good idea to assume that is the case. A baby growing slowly or not gaining at all for a few weeks is not a disaster. Missing a coarctation of the aorta because one assumes the problem is insufficient milk intake can be.

The benefits of exclusive breastfeeding are many. The question then arises: is it worth supplementing the baby with artificial milk to get somewhat faster weight gain? This is a difficult clinical question to answer. If the baby gains 150 grams a week (20 grams or 2/3 of an ounce a day) from week 4 to week 8, will this baby suffer in the future because of this slower than "usually acceptable" weight gain? No, I don't think there is any evidence to suggest this. If the baby is content and gaining slowly, then all we need to do is make sure the mother gets the help and information to follow the Protocol to increase breastmilk intake by the Baby and keep an eye on the baby for possible medical problems that may become more obvious with time. Not that the presence of a medical problem is a reason to add supplementation, but we do need to make sure we are not missing anything.

Of course, other circumstances may make supplementation desirable. A baby who is content, active, and gaining slowly and steadily is one thing. A baby who is gaining slowly and steadily but is a miserable, unhappy, screaming baby is another thing. In that case, we would be tempted to do more. But is supplementation the only thing that can be done?

Domperidone

Domperidone is a peripheral dopamine antagonist. It has been used since the mid 1980's or even a little before to treat nausea, vomiting, gastric reflux and gastric motility problems (as often seen in diabetics). It also inhibits dopamine secretion from the nuclei in the hypothalamus, dopamine being an inhibitor of prolactin secretion from the pituitary. Thus, by inhibiting dopamine secretion, prolactin secretion is increased. We believe that this is how domperidone increases milk supply since prolactin stimulates production of milk by the alveolar cells of the breast.

The use of domperidone for increasing milk supply is an "off label" use of the drug. This does not mean it cannot be used for this reason. Any legitimate therapeutic reason for using a drug is legal in most countries. However, this means that the company that makes the drug does not support its use, in the case of domperidone, for increasing milk supply.

Domperidone is not related to the drug cisapride, though many health professionals believe it is. It is used for the same reason as cisapride (gastric disturbances), but it is not in the same family and, except in very large doses used intravenously, has not caused death that has been reported.

Domperidone is far safer for mothers than a related drug, metoclopramide (Reglan, Maxeran). This is due to the fact that it seems not to pass the blood brain barrier in any significant amounts and thus the central nervous system effects (jitteriness, oculogyric crises, tardive dyskinesia, and depression) that one sees with metoclopramide are much rarer, if they occur at all, with domperidone than with metoclopramide. For this reason, domperidone can be used for months, even years, with few side effects in most patients.

The Federal Drug Administration (FDA) in the US does not feel the same way about the safety of domperidone. In June 2004, they issued a warning about breastfeeding women using domperidone and stated that they would urge custom officials to stop shipment of domperidone into the US. It is still possible to get domperidone in the US, as compounding pharmacies are not regulated by the FDA. But this makes it more complicated for breastfeeding women to obtain it, as many compounding pharmacies have complied with the FDA's absurd warning. My take on the FDA's statement follows (it was written in the summer of 2004):

As a pediatrician who deals now only with mothers and babies who are having difficulty with breastfeeding, I am very concerned about the warning about domperidone which was issued by the Federal Drug Administration in the US on June 7, 2004. It warns breastfeeding mothers about getting domperidone to enhance milk supply because it conceivably can cause cardiac arrhythmias.

The FDA has basically come up with a political statement. They seem really ticked off because people were going around using a drug that they have not approved. The deaths (and I believe there were two) occurred with intravenous domperidone, which is never used any more and has never been used for enhancing milk supply. It is likely that if this drug was given intravenously, the patients were sick with other problems as well, a confounding variable. Furthermore, unlike what the FDA has led people to believe, perhaps unintentionally, these are not new cases, but 2 decades old.

Why didn't they mention metoclopramide in their warning, which is far more dangerous (it can cause severe depression in oral doses, which domperidone does not), and is also being used off label to increase milk supply, but which, on the other hand, is available and approved for gastric motility problems in the US? Can it be that they are not concerned about the danger, but rather the threat to their authority? Here is part of a letter I received about metoclopramide and domperidone as a result of this to do about domperidone. "...my mother...is on domperidone for gastroparesis. She's 5 feet tall, and lost over 20 lbs...down to 82 lbs. And why is she on domperidone? Because she had depression and SEVERE panic attacks with the Reglan (metoclopramide). She was in and out of the senior psych ward all last spring. So my folks get domperidone from outside the US."

Why didn't they mention the danger to diabetics, if they are so concerned, for whom some endocrinologists in the US are prescribing domperidone for gastric paresis? Why specifically for breastfeeding women? Why not specifically for diabetics who are at much greater risk of cardiac arrhythmias than women of reproductive age?

Why did this warning come out almost exactly on the day that the National Breastfeeding Campaign was to begin in the US?

I have used domperidone in infants (for spitting up), but mostly to increase milk supply in women, probably well over 1000 women, without any more than mild headache, occasional menstrual irregularities, and mild abdominal cramping as side effects. I cannot say the same for metoclopramide which I saw causing severe CNS side effects, aside from depression.

I have personally seen two children die of Stevens-Johnson Syndrome after taking Septra. If I have seen two, how many have actually occurred in the US and Canada? Why are there no such warnings on Septra? I have, as a medical resident, seen at least one person die and several get severely ill after taking ASA from gastric bleeding. In overdose, many children have died and many have become seriously ill over the years because of ASA. Why is there no such warning on aspirin?

Many women have died and many more have been severely injured from taking the birth control pill. Why is it not banned?

The issue comes up about providing a drug for women in good health and that we should not be treating healthy women with a drug. I disagree. With all the talk about preventive medicine, when it actually comes down to trying to prevent illness, it is all lip service. The data are clear. Breastfeeding decreases the risk of breast cancer in the mother. For babies, it decreases the risk of diabetes (type I and II), obesity, hypertension, high LDL/HDL levels, otitis media, asthma, allergies, gastroenteritis, and in premature babies, necrotizing enterocolitis. The first 4 of these are all risk factors for atherosclerosis, the most significant degenerative disease in affluent societies and the biggest killer. The data are fairly clear that breastfeeding results in better cognitive development in children. The data are less clear, but suggestive, that breastfeeding decreases the risk of certain cancers in children (Hodgkin's and non Hodgkin's lymphoma, breast cancer in later life), multiple sclerosis, and inflammatory bowel disease.

Thus, we should do all that is reasonable to maintain and increase the success of woman who are breastfeeding. If this means that, in some cases, we use a drug that, in my experience of well over 1000 women, is safe with only minor side effects, we should have that option. Of course, there is no such thing as a drug which never causes side effects, and there are probably very few approved drugs (yes, even approved drugs) out there that haven't killed someone, but if one weighs the risk against the benefits, domperidone can do much good. I will continue to prescribe domperidone to women when I feel it will be useful. It's a shame, though, for women in the US to be deprived of this drug. The FDA says that it will monitor the border to make sure none gets through. Good for them. With heroine and cocaine getting through their borders as through a sieve, it's great that the US can now be sure that their borders are safe against an influx of the dreaded domperidone. What a waste of manpower! What a waste!

I would urge all practitioners to help mothers do the best for their children and use domperidone for increasing milk supply when this becomes necessary. Breastfeeding is important to the health of the mother and baby. We should act in consequence.

The dose of domperidone

According to the package insert, the maximum dose of domperidone to use is 20 mg four times a day. However, this is the dose for gastric problems. The dose to increase breastmilk production is generally greater than for gastric problems. However, gastroenterologists sometimes use significantly higher doses for gastric problems when they do not respond to the usual dose. For example, some patients take 40 mg 3 times a day. For increasing milk supply, we start with 30 mg 3 times a day. Occasionally, we have gone as high as 40 mg 4 times a day.

Using domperidone

It is vital to recognize that the problem of poor weight gain is frequently *not* simply a question of not enough production. True, the milk production does decrease over time if the baby does not breastfeed well. Nevertheless, we have seen many hundreds of babies whose mothers had more than ample milk supplies fail to gain adequately. A baby who does not latch on well has difficulty getting the milk that is there. That is simple.

Thus, it is crucial that before using domperidone, or at least, at the same time as starting domperidone, the first steps of the Protocol to Increase Breastmilk Intake by the Baby be shown the mother and the skills to follow the Protocol be taught her and her partner (if possible).

As a reminder, those steps are:

Protocol to Increase Breastmilk Intake by the Baby

1. Help the mother achieve the best latch possible.

2. Teach the mother how to know a baby is getting milk well.

3. When the baby is no longer drinking, use compression to keep the flow of milk up.

4. When the baby no longer drinks from the first side, offer the second, and repeat.

5. Going back to the first side again can be helpful, if the baby still drinks.

It seems that domperidone does not work particularly well in the first weeks (say 4 or 5 weeks) after the baby's birth. This may be because prolactin levels in the mother are already quite high during these first weeks, so that using domperidone is whipping a pituitary gland that is already working flat out. Generally, we tend not to start domperidone during the first month because despite warning mothers of its tendency not to be effective in the first few weeks, many got discouraged using it, and stopped using it before it had a chance to work. And because of this, some stopped breastfeeding.

One exception to the above is the situation of breast reduction. We have, because of the experience of others, including nursing mothers, started women with breast reduction on domperidone from the day of birth of the baby. There is no evidence, except anecdotal evidence, that this helps. Since the risk of insufficient milk supply is a serious one in women with this type of breast surgery, it seems worthwhile trying this approach.

It is not of value, however, to start domperidone during the pregnancy. Not only may there be unexpected side effects in the baby, though none have been described (the baby gets much more domperidone during pregnancy than during breastfeeding), it just won't do any good. It is better not to use a drug if it doesn't do any good and may do harm.

Domperidone tends to work best for women who once had a good milk supply but, for some reason, the milk supply decreased. Again, it is vital that the mother be following the Protocol to Increase Breastmilk Intake by the Baby and domperidone be *added* as part of the therapeutic approach.

How long does it take before domperidone starts to work? It usually starts fairly quickly, within a few days to a week, but sometimes the effect is delayed for a month or two. One should give it a trial for at least a month before saying it didn't work, but the dose can also be increased if necessary. After a week or two of little or no effect with our usual 30 mg tid, we will usually raise the dose to 40 mg tid. If that doesn't work, we will go up to a maximum 40 mg qid. These latter, higher doses are usually not necessary, however. We tend to use them more often, as we tend to see the most difficult cases, just as any speciality clinic will see the most difficult cases.

The idea, of course, is eventually to stop the domperidone. When to stop it is difficult to judge sometimes. Obviously, if the baby is breastfeeding exclusively and gaining weight well, it would be worth trying to wean the mother off the domperidone. Generally, we suggest dropping the dose slowly over several weeks. This may not be necessary, but I think it is. We ask the mother to drop a pill a day each week. Thus, if the mother is taking 30 mg tid, she can start taking 20 mg in the morning, 30 mg midday, and 30 mg in the evening. If the milk supply remains good and the baby continues feeding well, then mother drops another pill for a week, so she can take 20 mg in the morning, 20 mg at midday and 30 mg in the evening, and so on. At some point, either the mother will be down to no domperidone, which is great, or the milk supply will start to decrease. If the milk supply decreases, the mother can increase her dose to the previous effective number of pills and stay there for a few weeks before trying again to eliminate the domperidone. Some mothers will manage weaning the domperidone very well. Some will require domperidone as long as the baby is exclusively breastfeeding, but can either eliminate domperidone or decrease the dose significantly once the baby is taking solids. However, it should be remembered that babies like fast flow. If the milk supply decreases, milk flow may decrease and the baby may not be content at the breast even if the reduced milk supply is quite adequate for the needs of the baby.

If that occurs, there are three options. One is to increase the domperidone dose. The second is to give the baby some solid food before putting the baby to the breast. The baby should not be given so much he will be satiated and not want to breastfeed, but he should get enough so he is not ravenous when he goes to the breast. The third option is both of the above. One option does not exclude the other.

What if supplementation is necessary?

If, after all is done above, the baby needs to be supplemented because of poor weight gain, the best way of supplementing is with a lactation aid if the baby is under 4 to 6 months of age. After this time, the baby can be supplemented with food with milk mixed in with it. If done properly, using the lactation aid is easy and, in fact, takes less time than supplementing the baby otherwise. It is better than supplementing with a bottle, a syringe, an eyedropper, or a cup for the following reasons:

- Babies learn to breastfeed *by breastfeeding.*

- Mothers learn to breastfeed *by breastfeeding.*

- The baby continues to get milk from the breast, even during the actual supplementation.

- The baby will not reject the breast, which is very possible if you supplement the baby off the breast (yes, nipple confusion does exist, but it's not the baby who is confused).

- **There is more to breastfeeding than breastmilk.** Even some lactation specialists don't seem to understand this point. This is a consequence of our bottle feeding mentality, but also a disregarding of the emotional side of breastfeeding.

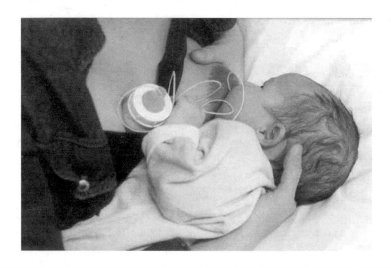

Mother supplementing with a lactation aid. Tube is 5French, 36 inches long. Bottle should be kept at about head level. Video clip of a mother using one can be seen at websites mentioned through or elsewhere in this chapter.

Once again, the importance of the latch is emphasized when using a lactation aid. The better the baby's latch, the less likely the mother will need to use the lactation aid. The better the baby's latch, the easier it is to use the lactation aid. The better the baby's latch, the sooner the mother can get rid of the lactation aid and the supplementation.

The lactation aid should be introduced only after the baby has fed on both sides with the mother following the Protocol to Increase Breastmilk Intake by the Baby. Some lactation consultants suggest introducing it as soon as the baby starts nursing, but this makes no sense to me at all. It suggests to the mother that the baby is getting no milk even at the beginning of the feeding. Furthermore, there is the very strong possibility that the baby will get used to the very fast flow that will occur and refuse to even start breastfeeding without the lactation aid being present. I have seen this happen many times.

The mother should offer both breasts at least as long as the baby is doing a decent amount of drinking and then start the supplementation. The baby should be allowed to drink as much as he wants, not some fixed amount. As the baby gets more milk from the breast, the baby will take less of the supplement. No need to suggest, for example, 60 ml at each feeding. This also makes no sense. What if the baby wants 75 ml or even 120 ml? What if the baby wants only 30 ml? Mothers have more milk in the morning, generally. Thus the baby may take little or no supplement in the morning, but take much more than 60 ml in the evening. With the lactation aid, it is better to give a little supplement at each feeding, than to try to feed the baby on the breast only most of the time and then give a large amount of supplement in the evening. Many mothers do this so that the baby will sleep better, but if the baby takes approximately 50 ml at each feeding 8 times a day, this is better than the baby taking 400 ml in two feedings in the evening. By giving some supplement at each feeding, each feeding is more effective and the mother has more time between feedings, which, in addition to allowing her some breathing space, also allows her breasts to "fill up more," so that the next feeding is better as well.

Over the weeks, if things go as we hope, the mother will use less and less supplement, automatically, and the baby will continue to breastfeed and get more and more milk from the breast. Some mothers will be able to breastfeed exclusively within a few weeks, some in even less time. Some mothers will never be able to do without the lactation aid. Is this a reason to switch to a bottle? No, babies of 4 months can reject the breast, too, if they start to get bottles.

In fact, if the baby is still getting supplemented by 4 months of age, I will usually suggest the mother add solids in a bid to get rid of the supplement. Of course, the mother can add previously expressed breastmilk or formula to the baby's solids (there is no need to drink the milk). As the baby gets more and more solids and milk by spoon, the baby will need less and less supplement in the lactation aid. Again, weaning from the supplement is done according to the baby's needs.

The issue of the baby fussing at the breast if the flow is slow is relevant here as well. Sometimes, it is worth giving the baby some solids before putting him to the breast so that he is not ravenous and won't mind the slower flow.

Many people have many strange ideas about the lactation aid. I will try to address these ideas now:

The lactation aid is difficult to use:

Well, some mothers find it difficult, others do not. Using the lactation aid easily comes with practice. Of course, if mothers are not shown how to use it properly, it is difficult to use, just as any tool used improperly does not get the job done. See the video clip showing how to use the lactation aid at the websites www.gentlemothering.ca or www. breastfeedingonline.com. These websites also have a patient information sheet on how to use the lactation aid.

It takes too long to supplement this way:

This is not true. In fact, once the mother knows how to use it properly, it would take less time. But the better the latch, the easier the lactation aid is to use and the better placed the tube, the faster the flow through it. It should not take an hour to get 60 ml of supplement into the baby. If that's what is happening, something is wrong. The latch or the position of the tube, or both, need fixing.

Mothers do have a tendency to try to squeeze the last drop out of the breast before introducing the lactation aid. This is not necessary and can result in the baby being on the breast for very long periods of time. It is not necessary to worry about trying to "empty the breast" because the baby will get that milk in any case since the baby is still on the breast and breastfeeding when using a lactation aid.

You can't use the lactation aid in public:

Why not? Too difficult to explain? Do we not hear how many mothers feel they are being judged if they are not breastfeeding? Well, this is a way to show the mother is trying. "For various reasons, I am not producing enough milk, but I want my baby to breastfeed. See how well he's doing, much better than a few weeks ago when he was starting to refuse the breast because of the bottles I was giving him."

I think these concerns are more often the result of the health care providers' lack of experience or perhaps lack of comfort with the lactation aid. This is a shame because supplementing the baby at the breast is the best way to supplement while maintaining breastfeeding.

Solving milk supply problems:

While milk supply problems can be complex and frustrating, by following the steps outlined here, most can be solved. It is also important to remember that some breastfeeding is better than none. Mothers who do not produce enough milk to breastfeed exclusively, even after following all the suggestions given here, can still breastfeed. They may need to supplement, but they can still breastfeed, and their babies will benefit tremendously when they do.

References

Breast Surgery

Kakagia D, Tripsiannis G, Tsoutsos D. Breastfeeding after reduction mammoplasty. *Ann Plast Surg* 2005 Oct;55(4):343-5.

Hefter W, Lindholm P, Elvenes OP. Lactation and breastfeeding ability following lateral pedicle mammoplasty. *Br J Plast Surg* 2003 Dec; 56(8):746-51.

Marshall DR, Callan PP, Nicholson W. Breastfeeding after reduction mammaplasty. *Br J Plastic Surg* 1994;47:167-9.

Scott-Conner CEH, Schorr SJ. The diagnosis and management of breast problems during pregnancy and lactation. *Am J Surg* 1995;170:401-5.

Hurst NM. Lactation after augmentation mammoplasty. *Obstet Gynecol* 1996;87:30-4.

Retained Placental Fragments

Byrne E. Breastmilk oversupply despite retained placental fragment. *J Hum Lact.* 1992 Sep;8 (3):52-3.

Sodium in Milk

Abu-Salah O. High breast milk sodium concentration resulting in neonatal hypernatraemic dehydration. *East Mediterr Health J.* 2001 Jul-Sep; 7 (4-5)841-3.

Humenick SS, Hill PD, Thompson J, Hart AM. Breast milk sodium as a predictor of breastfeeding patterns. *Can J Nurs Res.* 1998 Fall; 30(3):67-81.

Sofer S, Ben-Ezer D, Dagan R. Early severe dehydration in young breastfed newborn infants. *Isr J Med Sci* 1993;29:85-9.

Morton JA. The clinical usefulness of breastmilk sodium in the assessment of lactogenesis. *Pediatrics* 1994;93:802-6.

Soskolne EI, Schumacher R, Fyock C, Young ML, Schork A. The effect of early discharge and other factors on readmission rates of newborns. *Arch Pediatr Adolesc Med* 1995;150:373-9.

Livingstone VH, Willis CE, Abdel-Wareth LO, Thiessen P. Lockitch G. Neonatal hypernatremic dehydration associated with breastfeeding malnutrition: a retrospective survey. *Can Med Assoc J* 2000;162:647-52.

Sheehan's Syndrome

Feinberg EC, Molitch ME, Endres LK, Peaceman AM. The incidence of Sheehan's syndrome after obstetric hemorrhage. *Fertil Steril.* 2005 Oct;84(4):975-9.

Oral Contraceptives

WHO task force on oral contraceptives, special programme of research, development and research training in human reproduction. Effect of hormonal contraceptives on breastmilk composition and infant growth. *Studies in Family Planning* 1988;19:361-9.

Fraser IS. A review of the use of progesterone only minipills for contraception during lactation. *Reprod Fertil Dev* 1991;3:245-54.

Visness CM, Rivera R. Progestin only pill use and pill switching during breastfeeding. (editorial). *Contraception* 1995;51:279-81.

Guthmann RA, Bang J, Nashelsky J. Combined oral contraceptives for mothers who are breastfeeding. *Am Fam Physician* 2005 Oct 1;72(7):1303-4.

Insufficient Breast Tissue

Neifert MR, Seacat JM, Jobe WE. Lactation failure due to insufficient glandular development of the breast. *Pediatrics* 1985 Nov; 76(5):823-8.

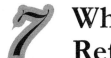

When the Baby Refuses to Latch On

One of the most frustrating situations for a new mother occurs when her baby simply refuses to latch on at all. It is a very emotional experience for the mother – she begins to worry first that her baby will starve, and secondly that her baby is in some way rejecting *her* as a mother. And of course mothers in the early days and weeks after giving birth are quite emotional and vulnerable even when everything is going smoothly. So it is important that situations like this are dealt with sensitively. You want to reassure the mother and give her confidence that her baby will, in time, learn to breastfeed.

Why would a baby refuse to take the breast?

Breastfeeding is a biologically normal and essential behavior, so the baby who won't breastfeed is not just a variation of normal. I have heard nurses say "Oh, some babies just don't want to breastfeed, they want the bottle" – and they were talking about newborns. This makes no sense. There is no inborn biological desire to be bottlefed. Babies who refuse the breast do so for a reason - in fact, often there is a combination of reasons. For example, a baby might latch on even with a tight frenulum if no other factors come into play, but if, for example, he is also given bottles early on, this additional factor may cause him to resist going to the breast.

Some examples:

1. If the mother's nipples are particularly large or inverted or flat, these nipple variations make latching on more difficult, though not usually impossible.

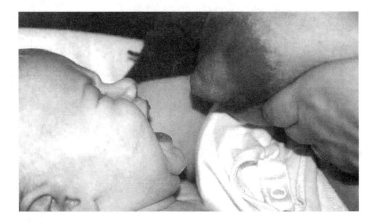

A very large nipple. The baby has difficulty latching on properly because of the size of the nipple, but he did eventually get it.

2. Some babies are unwilling to nurse or suck poorly as a result of medication they received during labor. Narcotic pain-relievers are responsible for many such situations, and meperidine (Demerol) is particularly bad as it stays in the baby's blood for a long time and affects the way he sucks for several days. I believe we are seeing more and more babies refusing the breast when the mother received morphine in an epidural (more so than with epidurals not containing morphine), but any medication from an epidural definitely does get into the mother's blood and thus into the baby (through the placenta) before he is born. These babies often go to the breast without protesting and may even take the nipple into their mouths, but then don't seem to know what to do next.

3. Vigorous suctioning at birth may result in babies not sucking properly and not wanting to latch on. Some will close their mouths tightly and resist any attempts to encourage them to open wide for the breast, acting as though they are afraid that letting anything in will mean more suctioning. (Of course, with a bottle you can force the nipple in – and doing that a few times may increase the baby's resistance still further.) There is no need to suction a healthy, full term baby at birth.

4. Abnormalities of the baby's mouth may result in the baby's not latching on. Cleft palate, but *not* usually cleft lip, causes severe difficulties in latching on. Sometimes the cleft palate is not obvious, affecting only the soft palate. Whenever a baby is having latching difficulties, a thorough examination should be done to rule out abnormalities of the mouth and palate.

5. A tight lingual frenulum may result in a baby having difficulty latching on because he cannot extend his tongue to properly cup the breast. This is not, strictly speaking, considered an abnormality, and thus, many physicians do not believe that it can interfere with breastfeeding, but they are misinformed.

6. A baby learns to breastfeed by breastfeeding. Artificial nipples interfere with how the baby takes the breast. Babies are not stupid. If they get slow flow from the breast (as is expected in the first few days of life) and rapid flow from the bottle, they will *not* be confused—many will figure it out quite quickly. They may then refuse to latch on to the breast at all.

However, one of the most common causes of babies' refusing to latch on arises from the **misguided** belief that babies in the first few days must breastfeed every 3 hours or on some other insane sort of schedule. This results in anxiety on the part of the staff when a baby has not fed, for example, for three hours after birth, which results, frequently, in babies being forcibly pushed into the breast when they are not ready yet to feed. When the baby's face is forced into the breast and kept there by force when the baby is not interested or ready, we should not be surprised that some babies develop an aversion to the breast. When, thanks to this misguided and forceful approach, the baby pushes away from the breast and refuses to nurse, panic often sets in and out of concern that "the baby *must* be fed," alternative feeding methods (the worst of which is the bottle) are quickly introduced, making the situation even worse. Soon the baby associates the breast with forceful handling and anxiety on the part of his mother and the staff, while the bottle becomes the reliable source of food, usually given much more calmly.

There is *no* evidence that a healthy full term newborn must feed every three hours during the first few days. There is *no* evidence that they will develop **low blood sugar** if they don't feed every three hours (the whole issue of low blood sugar has become a mass hysteria in newborn nurseries which, like all hysterias, results from a grain of truth, perhaps, but actually causes more problems than it prevents, including the problem of many babies getting formula when they don't need it, and being separated from their mothers when they don't need to be, and not latching on).

Babies should be skin-to-skin with their mothers most of 24 hours a day. When they are ready, most will start looking for the breast. Having the baby with the mother skin-to-skin immediately after birth and allowing the baby and the mother the time to "find" each other will prevent most situations of the baby not latching on. Mother and baby skin-to-skin will also keep the baby as warm as being under a heating lamp. And the mother will also feel relaxed and well rested with her new baby close to her.

What happens too often is that the mother and baby are given maybe five minutes together, and if the baby isn't feeding by the end of that time, everyone gets impatient. The mother and baby should be together until the baby latches on, without pressure and without time limits.

But the baby is not latching on! He'll starve!

Okay, so how long can we wait? There is no obvious answer to that. Certainly, if the baby has shown no interest in nursing or feeding by 12 to 24 hours after birth, it may be worthwhile to do something, *mostly because hospital policies usually require the mother to be discharged by 24 to 48 hours*. What can be done?

1. The mother should start expressing her milk and that milk (colostrum), either alone, or mixed with sugar water, should be fed to the baby, preferably by finger feeding. If it is difficult to get colostrum (often hand expression works better than a pump in the first few days), then sugar water alone is fine for the first few days. With finger feeding, most babies will start sucking, and many will wake up enough to attempt going to the breast. As soon as the baby is sucking well, which, in most cases takes no more than a minute or two, finger feeding should be stopped and the baby tried at the breast. Finger feeding is essentially a procedure to prepare the baby to take the breast, not primarily a method to avoid the bottle, though it will do that,

too. Therefore, it is done *before* attempting the baby at the breast to prepare him to take the breast.

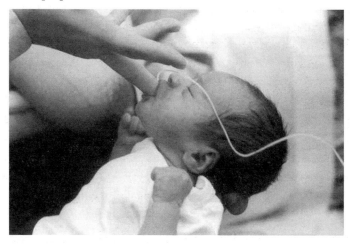

Finger feeding. The finger should be the largest with which the mother is comfortable and should be held flat in the baby's mouth so his tongue is brought forward and kept down.

2. Before discharge, early competent help needs to be arranged so that the mother and baby are getting help by day four or five at the latest. Many babies who do not latch on in the first few days will latch on beautifully once the mother's milk supply has increased substantially as it usually does around day 3 or 4. Getting help at this time avoids the negative associations with the breast that many babies develop as time goes on.

3. A nipple shield started before the mother's milk becomes abundant (day 4 to 5) is **bad practice**. Starting a nipple shield before the mother's milk "comes in" is not giving time a chance to work. Furthermore, used improperly (as I see it often being used), a nipple shield may result in severe depletion of the milk supply.

4. Use the baby's natural instincts to find the breast and latch on. Those instincts don't disappear an hour or two after birth. Encourage the mother to rest in a comfortable, warm room with her baby skin-to-skin and allow him to seek out her breast on his

own. The skin-to-skin part is very important. A baby wrapped in a blanket being held by his mother who is fully dressed is not going to begin seeking the breast. If the baby has come to resist the breast because he's been forced or pushed at the breast, this opportunity to latch on independently may be all he needs. Sometimes, for babies who have become very aversive or tense at the breast, having mother and baby take a relaxing, warm bath together will do the trick. When both are feeling comfortable together in the tub, the baby's natural instincts to breastfeed are stimulated and often he will latch on beautifully.

5. If the baby is crying or upset, trying to get him to latch is unlikely to work. Take some steps to calm the baby first. If he is crying even partially out of hunger, giving him some milk may be the best way to help him settle enough that he'll be willing to take the breast.

The baby is now five days old and still won't latch on. What do we do now?

First of all, don't be discouraged. Many babies who do not latch on in the early days or weeks will eventually come to the breast. Yes, it is better and easier if the baby latches on more quickly, but mothers often need to be reassured that most babies will eventually learn to breastfeed.

The single most important factor influencing whether or not the baby latches on is the mother's developing a good milk supply. If the mother's supply is abundant, most babies will latch on by 4 to 8 weeks of life even when many things have gone wrong in the beginning.

It is more important for the mother to build up and maintain a good milk supply than avoid a bottle. The bottle interferes. It is better if the parents use other methods (such as a cup) if they can, but many mothers will choose to use a bottle because it seems easier to them (and their families who may be helping them). In most cases the baby can still be taught to breastfeed.

At times when the baby is calm but showing early cues for feeding such as putting his hands to his mouth, smacking his lips, and turning his head towards the breast, the mother should carefully position the baby and help him to latch. As the baby comes onto the breast, she should compress her breast *so that the baby gets a gush of milk* right away. *Try the baby on the breast* he seems to prefer, or the breast that has more milk, *not the breast he resists more.*

If the baby latches on, he will start sucking and start drinking, and the mother can continue to use breast compression to help him get more milk easily.

If the baby doesn't latch on, the mother shouldn't try to force him to stay on the breast; **it won't work**. He will either get hysterical or "go limp." Have the mother move him away from the breast, perhaps bringing him up to her shoulder and gently patting his back to calm him, then watch for the baby to show signs of readiness before you start again. Often the baby who is held up against the mother's shoulder will instinctively try to move to the side and down his mother's body to seek the breast. This is an ideal moment to try offering the breast again. It is better to offer the breast, then move away, perhaps walking around the room with the baby and patting his back, then offer the breast again, several times, calming the baby each time, than to push him into the breast when he hasn't latched on.

If the baby continues to refuse or resist the breast, don't keep at it until he's angry. Try finger feeding a few seconds to a minute or two, and then try the breast again, perhaps on the other side. Finger feeding is to prepare the baby to take the breast, not primarily to avoid a bottle. If the baby is very hungry, the mother may have to give a little more supplement (breastmilk is the best supplement), so that he'll calm enough to work on learning to take the breast.

If the baby still doesn't latch on, the mother should finish the feeding with whatever method she finds easiest.

Using a lactation aid at the breast may be helpful, but often requires an extra hand.

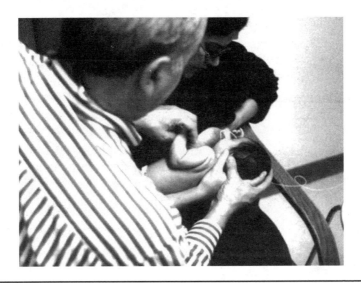

Getting the baby latched on with the lactation aid. The extra flow convinces the baby this is a good place to eat. Note that both our hands on not very well placed.

At about two weeks after birth, a change in what the mother has been doing often seems to send a message to the baby that "there's more than one way to get milk." If the mother has been finger feeding the baby exclusively, sometimes a change to a cup or bottle will help. If the baby has been bottle feeding, it may help to try finger feeding at least for a short time before trying the baby at the breast. Sometimes introducing a nipple shield at this point will do the trick and encourage the baby to latch. Another good time to try these, if the baby is still not latching, is around six weeks.

How to maintain and increase milk supply

Encourage the mother to express her milk as often as is practical, but if possible 8 times a day, using a high-quality, reliable pump that expresses both breasts at the same time. Using compression while pumping increases the efficiency of pumping and increases the milk supply (another hand is helpful, but mothers have rigged up the pump so that they don't have to hold onto the tubing or flanges while pumping and thus can compress without help).

Even the best pump is less effective than a baby who is nursing well, so the mother may need additional help to maintain good milk production. Fenugreek and blessed thistle (3 capsules 3 times a day - see chapter 6, page 131) can help increase milk flow, as can the prescription medication domperidone. In fact, we will almost always use the herbs to help with milk flow even if the mother has a good milk supply (enough so the mother does not need formula to keep the baby happy and growing). We often use domperidone even if the mother's milk supply is abundant, because it is more consistently reliable than the herbs.

Be prepared to give the mother lots of encouragement. Referral to a breastfeeding support group (such as La Leche League) may be very helpful. The mother needs to know that the baby is not rejecting her or rejecting her breasts, and that many babies who have initially refused to latch or had other latch difficulties do eventually learn to breastfeed beautifully and continue for many months or years.

References

Skin to Skin and Baby's Temperature

Christensson K, Siles C, Moreno L, Belaustequi A, De La Fuente P, Lagercrantz H, Puyol P, Winberg J. Temperature, metabolic adaptation and crying in healthy fullterm newborns cared for skin-to-skin or in a cot. *Acta Pediatr* 1992;81:488-93.

Jansson UM, Mustafa T, Khan MA, Lindblad BS, Widstrom AM. The effects of medically-oriented routines on prefeeding behaviour and body temperature in newborn infants. *J Trop Pediatr* 1995;41:360-3.

Christensson K. Fathers can effectively achieve heat conservation in healthy newborn infants. *Acta Paediatr* 1996;85:1354-60.

Christensson K, Bhat GJ, Amadi BC, Eriksson B, Höjer B. Randomised study of skin to skin versus incubator care for rewarming low risk hypothermic neonates. *Lancet* 1998;352:1115.

Effects of Labor Medications

Nissen E, Widstrom AM, Lilja G, Matthiesen AS, Uvnas-Moberg K, Jacobsson G, Boreus LO. Effects of routinely given pethidine during labour on infants' developing breastfeeding behaviour. Effects of dose - delivery time interval and various concentrations of pethidine/norpethidine in cord plasma. *Acta Paediatr* 1997;86:201-8.

Lie B, Juul J. Effect of epidural vs general anaesthetic on breastfeeding. *Acta Obstet Gynecol Scand* 1988;67:207-9.

Hypoglycemia

Williams AF. Hypoglycaemia of the newborn: a review of the literature. *World Health Organization*, Geneva. 1997.

Healing Sore and Damaged Nipples

Sore nipples are most commonly caused by one or both of two causes. **Either the baby is not positioned and latched properly or the baby is not suckling properly, or both.** These two things are naturally related as a baby's sucking problems may be caused by a poor latch, and a poor latch may be caused by an anatomical problem in the baby (such as a tongue-tie) which affects his sucking. There are, of course, other possible causes.

Mothers are encouraged and reassured when they learn that once the baby's latch is improved, their nipples will usually immediately feel less painful and begin healing. It is not necessary to wean temporarily to allow the nipples to heal – when the latch is correct, the nipples will not be compressed in baby's mouth and the pain will be significantly reduced. I've seen nipples that looked like raw hamburger and others that were more blister than nipple, and both types healed surprisingly quickly once the latch was improved.

It is not necessary to stop breastfeeding in order for the nipples to heal. In fact, a temporary weaning from the breast may lead to more problems. The baby still needs to be fed, after all, and often this means giving the baby bottles or using some other technique such as finger-feeding. If the baby's latch was not good to begin with (and therefore causing sore nipples), a few days of bottle-feeding may well make the baby's latch even worse when he returns to the breast. The mother's nipples may heal during the time the baby is not at the breast, only to be damaged even more once the baby returns to breastfeeding (if he will – some babies in this situation will simply decide that they prefer the bottle and refuse the breast altogether). Also, the mother will need to pump to provide milk for her baby (and to ensure her own comfort) and this can cause more nipple soreness as well. Furthermore, pumping is expensive if the mother rents or buys a pump and involves a fair amount of work. Taking a baby off the breast for any reason should be a last resort only. When I hear that a mother was advised to take the baby off the breast for a "nipple holiday" when the baby is 2 or 3 or even 4 or 5 days old, I know that this was not done as a last resort, but only because the mother had poor help.

Clearly, the first and most important step is to improve the baby's latch. Sometimes it takes only a small change in the baby's positioning, in the way the mother positions her hands, or in the timing of the mother's movements to make a huge difference in the effectiveness of the latch. Often, this is enough to immediately reduce the pain the mother has been experiencing and she is able to breastfeed much more comfortably.

It's also important to evaluate what is going on inside the baby's mouth. If the positioning seems good but the nipples are still being damaged, check for tongue-tie or other problems with the way the baby uses his tongue. Once these problems are corrected and the baby's suckling improves, the mother's nipples will start to heal.

However, sometimes the nipples have already been significantly damaged and then the mother may need more help and support as her nipples heal.

Some strategies to help nipples heal:

1. Always remember that the best strategy is prevention. When mothers are helped to latch their babies on correctly right from the beginning, these problems can be avoided. It is not helpful to tell mothers that "it's okay if it just hurts for the first minute and then gets better." A baby can do a lot of damage in one minute of nursing incorrectly, multiplied by several feedings every day.

2. Nipples can be warmed and dried for short periods of time after each feeding using a hair dryer on low setting.

3. Nipples should be exposed to the air as much as possible.

4. When it is not possible to expose nipples to air, plastic dome-shaped breast shells (**not** nipple shields) can be worn to protect the nipples from rubbing against the mother's clothing. Nursing pads keep moisture against the nipple and may cause damage that

way. They also tend to stick to damaged nipples and peeling them off is very painful. If the mother is leaking a lot, she can wear a nursing pad over the breast shell.

5. The mother can take over-the-counter painkillers such as acetaminophen.

6. The mother can express a little hind milk at the end of the feeding and gently rub it over the nipple, allowing it to dry there. Using breastmilk this way is soothing and also helps prevent infections.

7. Ointments can sometimes be helpful. Only a small amount of ointment should be used and the mother should be told not to wash it off before feedings. (The act of washing off the ointment will only make her nipples more sore.)

8. Remind the mother that frequent washing of the breasts and nipples is more likely to be harmful than helpful. Normal daily bathing is plenty. She should avoid using soap on her nipples, just rinse them with warm water.

9. If the baby is gaining weight well, there is no good reason the baby *must* be fed on both breasts at each feeding. The mother may feel it is easier for her to handle the pain if she just feeds one breast at each feeding. Using breast compression may help the baby to get more milk more quickly. She may also benefit by using a lactation aid with expressed milk to enable the baby to get a full feeding at one breast.

If the mother feels she can't put the baby to the breast because of the pain, be sure she knows that her nipples will heal quickly – usually within three to five days – and that if she maintains her milk supply the baby should come back to the breast. Some mothers with very sore or damaged nipples find that pumping is also painful and do better with hand-expressing their milk.

Because this is a baby who is already having difficulties latching and suckling well, it is better if the baby not get artificial (bottle or pacifier) nipples during this brief, temporary break from breastfeeding. Use the technique called "finger feeding" or cup feeding. This is a last resort and taking a baby off the breast should not be taken lightly.

Nipple shields are not recommended for sore nipples because, although they *may* help temporarily, they usually do not, or they *seem* to help only because the baby is not getting much of the nipple in his mouth. They may also cut down the milk supply dramatically, and the baby may become fussy and not gain weight well. Once the baby is used to them, it may be very difficult to get the baby back onto the breast. In fact, many women who have tried nipple shields find that they do not help with soreness.

Mothers should also be aware that when their nipples are damaged or cracked, these provide an entry for bacteria and they may be more susceptible to breast infections and inflammation. That's another reason for her to be sure to "keep the milk moving" while the nipples are healing.

We now have been using what I call an "all purpose nipple ointment" for 6 years, and many others who work with breastfeeding mothers have also begun recommending it. It works very well, much of the time. This combination of 3 ingredients seems to help for many causes of sore nipples, including poor latch, *Candida* (yeast), dermatologic conditions, infections of the nipple with bacteria and possibly other causes as well. It is always good, however, to try to assure the best latch possible because improving the latch helps with *any* cause of pain.

All Purpose Nipple Ointment

Mupirocin 2% *ointment* (not cream): 15 grams
Betamethasone 0.1% *ointment* (not cream): 15 grams.
to which is added **miconazole powder** so that the final concentration is 2% miconazole. Sometimes it is helpful to add **ibuprofen powder** as well, so that the final concentration of ibuprofen is 2%.

This combination gives a total volume of approximately 30 grams. **Clotrimazole powder** to a final concentration of 2% may be substituted if miconazole powder is unavailable, but both exist (the pharmacist may have to order it in). I believe clotrimazole is not as good as miconazole, but I have no proof of that. Using powder gives a better concentration of antifungal agent (miconazole or clotrimazole) and the concentrations of the mupirocin and betamethasone remain higher.

It is best to get the prescription filled at a compounding pharmacy. Too many mothers have been told, for example, that there is no such thing a miconazole powder. Yes, it does exist.

You can find a list of compounding pharmacies in Canada and the US by clicking http://www.iacprx.org/ There, if you click on the red box, "Help me find a compounding pharmacist" you will get to a search page that lets you search by postal code or zip code.

References

Nikoderm VC, Danziger D, Gebka N, Gulmezoglu AM, Hofmeyr GJ. Do cabbage leaves prevent breast engorgement? A randomized controlled study. *Birth* 1993;20: 61-4.

McLachlan Z, Milne EJ, Lumley J, Walker BL. Ultrasound treatment for breast engorgement: a randomised double blind trail. *Breastfeeding Review* 1993;May: 316-20.

Hill PD, Humenick SS. The occurrence of breast engorgement. *J Hum Lact* 1994;10:79-86.

Humenick SS, Hill PD, Anderson MA. Breast engorgement: patterns and selected outcomes. *J Hum Lact* 1994;10:87-93.

Evans K, Evans R, Simmer K. Effect of the method of breastfeeding on breast engorgement, mastitis and infantile colic. *Acta Paediatr* 1995;84:849-52 (kept under Colic).

Woolridge MW. Aetiology of sore nipples. *Midwifery* 1986;2:172-7.

Ziemer MM, Pigeon JG. Skin changes and pain in the nipple during the first week of lactation. *JOGNN* 1993;22:247-56.

Kesaree N, Banapurmath CR, Banapurmath S, Shamanur K. Treatment of inverted nipples using a disposable syringe. *J Hum Lact* 1993;9:27-9.

The MAIN Trail Collaborative Group. Preparing for breastfeeding: treatment of inverted and non protractile nipples in pregnancy. *Midwifery* 1994;10:200-14.

Lavergne NA. Does application of tea bags to sore nipples while breastfeeding provide effective relief? *JOGNN* 1997;26;53-8.

Department of child and adolescent health and development, World Health Organization. Mastitis: causes and management. WHO document, WHO/FCH/CAH/00.13, Geneva, 2000.

Fetherston C. Mastitis in lactating women: physiology or pathology? *Breastfeeding Review* 2001;9(1):5-12.

Hall DMB, Renfrew MJ. Tongue tie. *Arch Dis Child* 2005;90:1211-1215.

The Premature Baby

While current hospital practices often make breastfeeding difficult for full term, healthy babies born uneventfully to mothers who are also in good health, the story is even worse for babies and mothers who don't quite fit this model. These babies are often separated from their mothers, usually for no good reason, and supplementation begins early and is given often and commonly by bottle before the baby is even offering the breast.

When it comes to the premature baby, the separation and the inappropriate methods of feeding become almost universal, usually for a much longer period of time than for any full term baby. As well, even though more health professionals are beginning to understand how interference with breastfeeding in the early days and weeks can damage the breastfeeding in a full term healthy baby, too many still accept that feeding the premature baby *requires* mother infant separation, delay of breastfeeding initiation, limitation of breastfeeding, and early use of artificial nipples. Indeed, unlike the now generally accepted notion that exclusive breastfeeding is appropriate and preferable to supplementation in the full term infant, many pediatricians and neonatologists do not accept that the premature baby can get adequate nutrition and grow appropriately on breastmilk alone. And breast*feeding*, actually feeding on the breast? Impossible!

It's not only possible but **better** for the premature baby to breastfeed and breastfeed exclusively, at least in the vast majority of cases. It's just that we've been going about the whole business in the wrong way. In a field (neonatology) where "evidence based medicine" is often invoked to criticize breastfeeding as the appropriate way of feeding premature babies, it is shocking to see how much evidence is simply ignored or disregarded with regard to breastfeeding. We have a substantial body of evidence showing that incubator care is inferior to Kangaroo Mother Care not only for getting babies breastfeeding earlier, but also in maintaining metabolic stability of the premature baby; that premature babies can begin breastfeeding much earlier than the "traditional" 34 weeks gestation, and that premature babies can breastfeed exclusively and achieve adequate growth. Why is this important data ignored? It is too often a matter, one can only conclude, of "we've always done it this way and we will continue to do it this way."

But just as the full term baby may not breastfeed well and get adequate intake of milk if he does not latch on properly, the same is true of the premature baby. Yes, of course, there are more challenges: the premature baby may have significant medical problems; the premature baby tends to have less well developed feeding reflexes; the premature baby is smaller, and it may be more difficult for the baby to get a large part of the breast into his mouth. These and other objections are true to a certain degree in many premature babies. However, just like full term babies, premature babies learn to breastfeed by breastfeeding, and they cannot learn to breastfeed while lying in an incubator.

Too often the attitude in special care units is that the staff is dealing with life-threatening illness and there is no time for breastfeeding. But helping the baby survive and helping the mother and baby learn to breastfeed are not mutually exclusive. The purpose of the special care unit is not only the immediate survival of the baby, but also the long term health and development of the baby. Breastfeeding does much to assure long term good health in the baby and prevents problems of attachment and bonding, which are common in premature babies and their families. Too often, the baby born prematurely is neglected once home, even abused, and part of the fault lies in the way we separate mothers and babies, making mothers feel unworthy and unimportant in our special care units while encouraging them to detach from their infants. Helping the mother achieve successful breastfeeding can prevent many such problems of attachment and bonding.

Kangaroo Mother Care: the standard of care for premature babies

Since the 1980's when Kangaroo Mother Care was found to result in fewer deaths and better breastfeeding success in premature babies in Columbia, the number of studies that have confirmed this has multiplied to show not only benefit for healthy prematures, but also prematures who require oxygen and even ventilation. In the words of Dr. Nils Bergmann, a neonatologist working in South Africa, the baby's "normal habitat" is skin-to-skin with the mother, not in an incubator. Babies separated from their mothers and left lying in incubators go into despair, and the experience is highly stressful for them with all the physical and health consequences you expect from putting this tiny baby under stress.

Indeed, studies over the years have shown that premature babies cared for skin-to-skin with the mother were better able to maintain their body temperatures and blood sugars. They were less likely to develop apneas and bradycardias. In other words, many of the reasons that premature babies are kept in incubators were actually shown to be invalid and that Kangaroo Mother Care was actually superior to the incubator in both preventing and treating these concerns. Of significant importance is the fact that premature babies cared for skin-to-skin are also more likely to latch on earlier to the breast, are more likely to latch on better (and thus learn to breastfeed well earlier), and more likely to leave the hospital breastfeeding exclusively. This gives them a better foundation for future health and growth.

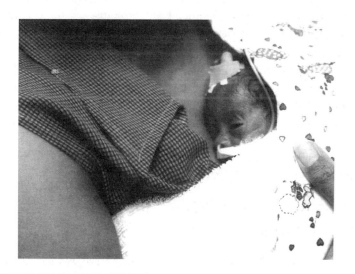

29 week gestation baby, Kangaroo mother care. The baby is better off here than in the incubator.

How early can premature babies go to the breast?

It has long been a rule of neonatal units that babies were not ready to start breastfeeding until they were at least 34 weeks gestation. This had to do with their "inability" to coordinate breathing, sucking, and swallowing with the danger of apneas, bradycardias, and aspiration. However, this rule was based on an inappropriate cohort, a bottle feeding cohort, and it is true that bottle feeding babies are more likely to have the above problems. But what is true for a bottle feeding baby is not necessarily true for the breastfeeding baby. Indeed, much of the difficulty that many health professionals and lay people have in understanding breastfeeding comes from the fact that we use the bottle feeding model as the model of normal, and then attempt to impose that model on the breastfeeding mother and baby. This is, in the old expression, comparing apples to oranges. It just doesn't work. The two are not the same.

In fact, work done in Sweden and elsewhere has shown us that premature babies can breastfeed well before 34 weeks gestation. Indeed, by encouraging Kangaroo Mother Care (not just an hour or two a day as is done in some places, but as many hours out of the day as possible), by allowing the baby free access to the breast and not just allowing feedings on a hospital-based schedule (this is an intrinsic part of Kangaroo Mother Care), and by encouraging the baby to go to the breast, premature babies in these places are not uncommonly achieving *full* breastfeeding by 33 weeks gestation, occasionally even earlier. This is in contrast to the situation in many North American hospitals, where in many special care units, the babies are not even yet "allowed" to go the breast for fear they are not ready.

In several special care units, babies are nuzzling the breast by 28 weeks gestation, and some are actually latching on not long after that. The photo shown here is of a 3 day old 31 week gestation baby who is breastfeeding well (not just sucking at the breast).

There is no reason, except "tradition" and adherence to inappropriate rules regarding premature babies, that this cannot be done everywhere.

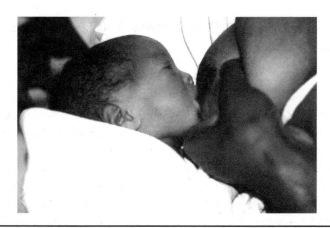

3 day old 31 week gestation baby. Breastfeeding with beautiful pauses in the chin. Note the asymmetric latch. (Mother did this without being shown. She is also using compression without having been shown.)

Premature babies, bottles, pacifiers and nipple shields

In many special care units, pacifiers are given to premature babies from very early on with the belief that they will grow faster and "learn to suck" better, and bottles are often foisted onto parents to "get the baby feeding faster." In addition, in some units, nipple shields are started early because of the belief that premature babies breastfeed better and get more milk when they use a special premature nipple shield.

I believe the above is unfortunate and has more to do with trying to get the baby out of the hospital faster, thus saving money, rather than serving the long-term good of the babies and their mothers. Breastfeeding is sacrificed, as it often is, to expediency.

With widespread Kangaroo Mother Care, with abandoning the "can't breastfeed until 34 weeks gestation" rule, and with good help for mothers in helping their premature babies achieve a good latch, bottles, pacifiers, and nipple shields should not be necessary in most cases.

One mother I saw had a 32-week premature baby. She was staying in the "care-by-parent" room attached to the special care nursery and was available for him 24 hours a day. The hospital staff wanted her to give the baby a pacifier because sucking on the pacifier would reduce his stress and help him to grow better. The mother asked why she could not just hold the baby skin-to-skin and let him suckle at her breast when he wanted to. No, the nurse told her, that would be too stressful for the baby because he'd get milk and have to coordinate sucking and swallowing. Fine, the mother said, I can pump first and the baby can suckle on the almost-emptied breast. The nurse still objected, saying that being held by his mother would be more stressful for the baby because it would overstimulate him – he needed to be alone in his incubator.

The mother pointed out that since the baby was hooked up to monitors, it would be easy to assess whether being held skin-to-skin actually stressed him. She wrote down the respiration rate, heart rate, etc. that the monitors showed when the baby was in the incubator. Then she picked him up and put him against her bare chest. Not only was he not stressed, it was clear that his breathing, temperature, and other vital signs improved when he was skin-to-skin. Reluctantly, the hospital staff gave in.

This should not be a battle that individual mothers have to fight with nursery staff. Breastfeeding should be supported and encouraged as much as possible.

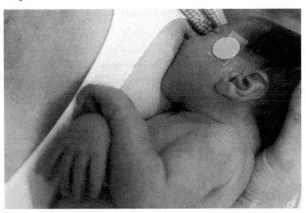

34 week gestation baby. Mother was told baby was not ready to put to breast yet. Latched on easily and breastfed beautifully and is now starting to sleep. Nose is a little too close to the breast, but it worked anyway.

What if the baby is feeding at the breast and needs a supplement? The whole question of how much a premature baby should take needs to be reviewed and confirmed by further research. A baby who has free access to the breast (Kangaroo Mother Care), who has received help in getting a good latch, who is not limited in the time "allowed" at the breast and who is not forced to feed on a three hour schedule may not need any supplement. How do we know how much breastmilk a baby of 31 weeks and weighing 1200 grams actually needs? The numbers usually given are based on an unproven premise (the baby needs to grow at intrauterine rates). There is some research to suggest that premature babies who grow very rapidly, usually on formula, are at a greater risk of health problems later in life. Perhaps this push for rapid growth is actually putting too much stress on the baby's system.

Furthermore, the expected weight gains are also based on breastmilk that has been "fortified." In some cases, "fortification" *may* be necessary, but in too many cases, one would more accurately call the process of adding "human milk fortifier" to breastmilk "dilution" of breastmilk.

But what if the baby really does need a supplement? Let us say that after the feeding, the baby cries and roots and is still hungry? Well, before going into supplementation, it is important to try to get the baby to latch on as well as possible. A baby who latches better gets more milk. The nipple shield has been justified because the baby gets more milk while using the nipple shield, but this can only mean that the baby's latch at the breast is better with the nipple shield than it is without. Does this mean that a better latch without the nipple shield is impractical? Not at all! Indeed, if the latch with the nipple shield is better than without it, that latch without a nipple shield has to be pretty awful, and it should be possible to do better. Furthermore, breast compression can be utilized to help the baby get more milk. Switching to the other breast once the baby no longer gets milk is also a good stratagem.

And what if the baby still shows he's hungry? Then a lactation aid can be used to supplement, but not before trying to get the baby to breastfeed better. There are several reasons to prefer such a measure to the bottle or any alternative feeding method not including the baby at the breast.

1. Babies, even premature babies, perhaps especially premature babies, learn to breastfeed by breastfeeding.

2. Mothers of premature babies, just as mothers of full term babies, learn to breastfeed by breastfeeding.

3. When using a lactation aid, the baby continues to get flow and continues breastfeeding. It is said that premature babies tire at the breast and thus need to be supplemented by nasogastric tube or bottle or cup, but this is false in most cases. True, if the baby needs oxygen or is in cardiac or respiratory insufficiency, he may not be able to maintain breastfeeding, but then he would not be able to maintain bottle feeding either. In general, premature babies "tire" at the breast for the same reason as full term babies, that is, because the flow of milk decreases. When the flow slows, babies tend to fall asleep at the breast. This is true for full term babies, in general, often until 6 or 8 weeks after birth. And this is true for premature babies as well. Keep up the flow of milk and the baby will keep feeding and stay awake quite well. Again, the key word here is *feeding* at the breast, not just sucking. If the baby is feeding at the breast, even with his eyes closed, this is fine. If there is concern, oxygen saturation of the baby can be followed while the baby feeds.

4. When the lactation aid is used, the baby continues to get milk from the breast even when being supplemented. This increases the mother's milk supply.

5. Babies will not usually reject the breast if not given artificial nipples. There is a huge controversy about whether "nipple confusion" exists. I cannot understand why this is controversial. Of course it exists, and it exists particularly when breastfeeding is most fragile - in other words, when a baby has a bad latch already or when the mother's milk supply is not abundant, use of artificial nipples is much more likely to cause a problem. Babies, even premature babies, are not stupid. If they get slow flow from the breast and rapid flow from a bottle, many will figure that out pretty quickly and prefer the bottle to the breast. It's important to consider how this affects the mother as well. A new mother whose baby appears to prefer the bottle to her

breast often feels rejected and discouraged. If she is already struggling to connect with her baby because of prematurity and separation, this may further damage the relationship.

6. There is much more to breastfeeding than breastmilk alone. This is a difficult statement to prove scientifically, but there is no question that the act of breastfeeding is much more than providing nutrition to the baby. Thus, even if the mother has very little milk, it is still better to have the baby supplemented at the breast than to say to a mother to feed the baby x minutes on each side and then give a bottle. Even if the baby does not refuse the breast, there is much more in the act of breastfeeding than the milk. In our society, this is often put down as "oh, you mean the bonding," as if that were of no import. But it is tremendously important. It is the foundation of the mother and child relationship. Unfortunately, too many health professionals do not recognize this as a valid issue and just don't see what the issue is exactly. Why is this mother insisting on putting the baby to the breast? They cannot understand.

Latching on the premature baby

The technique for latching on a premature baby is actually the same as that used for a full term baby – with a little added patience. Yes, it may take more time. Yes, the baby may not seem immediately interested. Yes, we have to give the baby nuzzling time and getting used to the idea time. But essentially, the approach is the same. In fact, I think the cross cradle hold used to describe how to latch on the full term baby was initially derived from the techniques of latching on the premature baby. The cross cradle hold allows the mother to support the premature baby's head more confidently, as the premature holds his head less well than a full term baby.

The baby's small size may mean that he needs a more asymmetric latch to get the maximum amount of milk. Help the mother to ensure that his chin is well under the breast and his nose is clear. Having the chin pressed well into the breast helps to stabilize it, although at times mothers may need to gently press against the chin with one finger to help the baby open as wide as he can and latch well. Compression may also help to give the baby the maximum amount of milk at each feeding.

A patient but persistent approach to breastfeeding will work with most premature babies. Even though they are tiny, the inborn breastfeeding instincts are there and just waiting to emerge if we give them a chance.

References

Risks of Not Breastfeeding (specific to the premature)

Carlson SE, Rhodes PG, Ferguson MG. **Docosahexaenoic acid status** of preterm infants at birth and following feeding with human milk or formula. *Am J Clin Nutr* 1986;44:798-804.

Morley R, Cole TJ, Powell R, Lucas A. Mother's choice to provide breastmilk and developmental outcome. *Arch Dis Child* 1988;63:1382-5.

Lucas A, Cole TJ. Breastmilk and neonatal necrotizing enterocolitis. *Lancet* 1990;336:1519-23.

Uauy RD, Birch DG, Birch EE, Tyson JE, Hoffman DR. Effect of dietary omega-3 fatty acids on **retinal function** of very low birth weight neonates. *Pediatr Res* 1990;28:485-92.

Lucas A, Morley R, Cole TJ, Lister G, Leeson-Payne C. Breastmilk and subsequent intelligence quotient in children born preterm. *Lancet* 1992;339:261-4.

Bishop NJ, Dahlenburg SL, Fewtrell MS, Morley R, Lucas A. Early diet of preterm infants and **bone mineralization** at age five years. *Acta Paediatr* 1996;85:230-6.

El-Mohandes AE, Picard MB, Simmens SJ, Keiser JF. Use of human milk in the intesive care nursery decreases the incidence of **nosocomial sepsis**. *J Perinatol* 1997;17:130-4.

Daniels L, Gibson R, Simmer K. Selenium status of preterm infants: the effect of postnatal age and method of feeding. *Acta Pædiatr* 1997;86:281-8.

Foreman-van Drongelen MMHP, van Houwelingen AC, Kester ADM, Hasaart THM, Blanco CE, Hornstra G. **Long-chain polyunsaturated fatty acids** in preterm infants: status at birth and its influence on postnatal levels. *J Pediatr* 1997;126:611-8.

Bier JB, Ferguson AE, Morales Y, Liebling JA, Oh W, Vohr BR. Breastfeeding infants who were extremely low birth weight. *Pediatrics* 1997;100:p e3.

Singhal A, Cole T, Lucas A. Early nutrition in preterm infants and later blood pressure: two cohorts after randomised trials. *Lancet* 2001;357:413-9.

Hylander MA, Strobino DM, Pezzullo JC, Dhanireddy R. Association of human milk feedings with a reduction in retinopathy of prematurity among very low birth weight infants. *J Perinatology* 2001;21:356-62.

Bier JB, Oliver T, Ferguson A, Vohr BR. Human milk reduces outpatient upper respiratory symptoms in premature infants during their first year of life. *J Perinatology* 2002;22:354-9.

Feldman R, Eidelman AI. Direct and indirect effects of breastmilk on the neurobehavioral and cognitive development of premature infants. *Dev Psychobiol* 2003;43:109.

McGuire W, Anthony MW. Donor human milk versus formula for preventing necrotising enterocolitis in preterm infants: systematic review. *Arch Dis Child Fetal Neonatal Ed* 2003;88:F11-F14.

Singhal A, Cole T, Lucas A. Breastmilk feeding and lipoprotein profile in adolescents born preterm: followup of a prospective randomised study. *Lancet* 2004;363:1571-8.

Rønnestad A, *et al*. Late onset septicemia in a Norwegian national cohort of extremely premature babies receiving very early full human milk feedings. *Pediatrics* 2005;215:e262-e268.

Singhal A, Cole TJ, Fewtrell M, *et al*. Is slower early growth beneficial for long term cardiovascular health? *Circulation* 2004;109:1108-13.

Singhal A, Fewtrell M, Cole TJ, Lucas A. Low nutrient intake and early growth for later insulin resistance in adolescents born preterm. *The Lancet* 2003;361 (March 29):1089-97.

Singhal A, Farooqi IS, O'Rahilly S *et al*. Early nutrition and leptin cencentrations in later life. *Am J Clin Nutr* 2002;75: 993-9.

Kangaroo Mother Care (prematures only)

Charpak N, Ruiz-Peláez JG, Figueroa Z, Charpak Y. Kangaroo mother versus traditional care for newborn infants <2000 grams: a randomized, controlled trial. *Pediatrics* 1997;100:682-8.

Cattaneo A, Davanzo R, Worku B, Surjono A, Echeverria M, Bedri A, *et al*. Kangaroo Mother Care for low birthweight infants: a randomized controlled trial in different settings. *Acta Pædiatr* 1998;87:976-85.

Fischer CB, Sontheimer D, Scheffer F, *et al.* Cardiorespiratory stability of premature boys and girls during kangaroo care. *Early Human Development* 1998;52:145-53.

Törnhage C-J, Stuge E, Lindberg T, Serenius F. First week kangaroo care in sick very preterm infants. *Acta Pædiatr* 1999;88:1402-4.

Furman L, Kennell J. Breastmilk and skin to skin kangaroo care for premature infants: avoiding bonding failure. *Acta Pædiatr* 2000;89:1280-3.

Föhe K, Kropf S, Avenarius S. Skin to skin contact improves gas exchange in premature. *J Perinatology* 2000;5:311-15.

Charpak N, Ruiz-Peláez JG, Figueroa Z, Charpak Y. A randomized, controlled trial of kangaroo mother care: results of follow-up at 1 year corrected age. *Pediatrics* 2001;108:1072-9.

Furman L, Minich N, Hack M. Correlates of lactation in mothers of very low birth weight infants. *Pediatrics* 2002;109(4) www.pediatrics.org/cgi/content/full/109/4/e57

Ohgi S, Fukuda M, Moriuchi T, *et al.* Comparison of kangaroo care and standard care: behavioural organization, development and temperament in health low birth weight infants through 1 year. *J Perinatology* 2002;22:374-9.

Feldman R, Weller A, Sirota L, Eidelman AI. Skin to skin contact (Kangaroo care) promotes self-regulation in premature infants: sleep-wake cyclicity, arousal modulation, and sustained exploration. *Dev Psychobiol* 2002;38:194-207.

Johnston CC, Stevens B, Pinelli J, Gibbins S, Filion F, Jack A, *et al.* Kangaroo care is effective in diminishing pain response in preterm infants. *Arch Pediatr Adolesc Med* 2003;157:1084-8.

Ruiz-Paláez JG. Charpak N, Cuervo LG. Kangaroo Mother Care, an example to follow from developing countries. *Br Med J* 2004;329:1179-82.

Bergman NJ, Linley LL, Fawcus SR. Randomized controlled trial of skin to skin contact from birth versus conventional incubator for physiological stabilization in 1200 to 2199 gram newborns. *Acta Pædiatr* 2004;93:779-85.

WHO document for skin to skin care (with many references): www.who.int/reproductivehealth/publications/kmc/kmctext.pdf.

Other

Hedberg Nyqvist K, Ewald U. Infant and maternal factors in the development of breastfeeding behaviour and breastfeeding outcome in preterm infants. *Acta Pædiatr* 1999;88:1194-1203. *(prematures can breastfeed)*

Marinelli KA, Burke GS, Dodd VL. A comparison of the safety of cup feedings and bottle feedings in premature infants whose mothers intend to breastfeed. *J Perinatology* 2001;21:350-5. *(babies more likely to desaturate during bottle feedings compared to cup feedings)*

Chan M, Nohara M, Chan BR, Curtis J, Chan GM. Lecithin decreases human milk fat loss during enteral pumping. *J Pediatr Gastroenterol Nutr* 2003;36:613-5.

O'Connor D, Jacobs J, Hall R, Adamkin D, Auestad N, *et al*. Growth and development of premature infants fed predominantly human milk, predominantly premature formula, or a combination of human milk and premature formula. *J Pediatr Gastroenterol Nutr* 2003;37:437-46.

Lubetsky R, Vasman N, Mimouni FB, Dollberg S. Energy expenditure in human milk versus formula fed preterm infants. *J Pediatr* 2003;143:750-3. *(human milk fed infants used less energy)*

Collins CT, Ryan P, Crowther CA, McPhee AJ, Patterson S, Hiller JE. Effects of bottles, cups and dummies on breastfeeding in premature infants: a randomised controlled study. *Br Med J* 2004;329:193-8. *(prematures fed with cups rather than bottles were more likely to leave hospital breastfeeding)*

Bishop NJ, Dahlenburg SL, Fewtrell MS, *et al*. Early diet of preterm infants and bone mineralization at age five years. *Acta Pædiatr* 1996;85:230-6.

Nutrient needs and feeding of premature babies. Statement of the Canadian Paediatric Society, 1995. (available at http://www.cps.ca/english/publications/Nutrition.htm)

Dslina A, Christensson K, Alfredsson L, *et al*. Continous feeding promotes gastroentestinal tolerance and growth in very low birth weight infants. *J Pediatr* 2005;147:43-49.

Nyqvist KH, Sjö P-O, Ewald U. The development of preterm infants' breastfeeding behaviour. *Early Hum Dev*. 1999;55:247-264.

Mizuno K, Ueda A. Changes in sucking performance from Nonnutritive sucking to Nutritive sucking during breast- and bottle-feeding. *Pediatr Res* 2006;59:728-31.

Gomes CF, Trezza EMC, Murade ECM, Padovani CR. Surface electromyography of facial muscles during natural and artificial feeding of infants. *J Pediatr (Rio J)* 2006;82(2):103-9.

10 Slow Weight Gain after Initial Adequate Gain

Usually, babies who gain weight well for the first few weeks will continue to gain weight well on breastfeeding alone until 6 months of age and sometimes for several months longer. Many continue to gain well on exclusive breastfeeding with no other liquids or solids until a year or more. Generally, I feel that babies should not be started on solid foods until they are showing readiness for eating by trying to grab food and put it into their mouths. This usually occurs around the middle of the first year.

However, for various reasons, some babies start not to gain weight well after an initially good weight gain. Of course, it is normal for the baby's rate of weight gain to decrease after the first few months, but these cases are babies who are gaining weight too slowly and sometimes not gaining at all. Some start to slow down too much by six weeks or so, some only around 4 or 5 months. We also see everything in between. We are now seeing more and more of these babies. I think this is because more and more mothers have been breastfeeding exclusively longer and longer. Unfortunately, too often the information they have received over their breastfeeding experience has not improved as much as one would like. The following case study is typical.

Case Study:

JW was born after a normal pregnancy and birth, the first live birth for a 33 year old mother. Breastfeeding commenced very well immediately after birth and no supplements or pacifiers were ever used in the hospital or after. The baby was born at 3.4 kg (7 lb 8 oz). According to the information the mother brought with her to our clinic, he weighed 3.3 kg (7 lb 4 oz) at one week of age, 4.5 kg (just under 10 lb) at one month, 5.7 kg (12 lb 9 oz) at two months of age. However, when the mother brought the baby to the family doctor at 3 months of age, he weighed only 5.9 kg (13 lb). Considering that perhaps the previous weight might be an error, the physician asked the mother to return with the baby when the baby was four months of age. At that point the baby weighed 5.9 kg again.

We saw the baby in the breastfeeding clinic when the baby was a few days over 4 months of age. In the history, the mother said she was not on the birth control pill or any other medication. The mother was certain that she was not pregnant, and she said she was not supplementing the baby, giving bottles, or using a pacifier. She stated that the baby would nurse about 8 times a day, twice between midnight and 6:00 a.m. The baby would spend only 3 or 4 minutes at most on the breast, and then would pull off and suck his hand. If she tried to put him back to the breast, he would fight the breast. If she offered the other breast, he would sometimes, but not always, take the second breast, but again only for a short period of time. After nursing for a short period of time, the baby would pull off and suck his hand again, apparently perfectly content.

Observation of the breastfeeding showed that the baby was sucking but actually drinking very little at the breast. He was very distractible while breastfeeding, pulling off the breast whenever anyone spoke. This exaggerated distractibility (most babies at this age are somewhat distractible) is very typical behavior for babies of this age when the milk supply has decreased.

One can tell when the baby is getting milk at the breast (rather than sucking without getting milk) by observing the baby's chin while he nurses. When a baby is getting milk (he is *not* getting milk just because he has the breast in his mouth and is making sucking movements), one can see a pause at the point of his chin after he opens to the maximum and before he closes his mouth (one suck is open mouth wide-->*pause*-->close mouth). We teach this to the mother by demonstrating this pause while the baby drinks at the breast. This **visible** pause **in the motion of the baby's chin** represents a mouthful of milk. The longer the pause, the more the baby got. Some of the video clips at www.breastfeedingonline. com, www.thebirthden.com/Newman.html or www.gentlemothering.ca show this pause very clearly. It was obvious from our observations of this baby feeding that he was not getting much milk.

Physical examination was unremarkable except that the baby was thin. He was alert and happy with no evidence of cardiac or any other disease. His weight was 5.88 kg on our scale.

A urinalysis was done just to be sure and was negative, though it was obvious that the baby wasn't getting milk at the breast in any significant amounts (from observation) and that the cause of the slow weight gain was inadequate intake, not illness in the baby. The mother had had her thyroid function checked by the family doctor, and it had come back within normal levels.

What might have caused this decrease in milk production? And what does latch have to do with it?

As mentioned in the introduction, this phenomenon is not rare in our clinic. We see easily 3 or 4 such mothers a month, but we deal through email and telephone with many more. Almost every day, I receive at least one email detailing how the baby was breastfeeding and gaining well, and then is no longer gaining and often no longer happy at the breast. Of course, it is difficult to say how common it is, since the population is very much skewed by the fact that we see only mothers and babies who are having problems. However, our experience has demonstrated that the following factors should be considered as possible causes of a late-onset decrease in milk supply:

1. **The mother has gone on a birth control pill.** This is one of the most common reasons we see or hear about. There is no doubt that hormonal contraceptives, particularly those containing estrogens may cause very significant decreases in the mother's milk supply, usually within a week or 10 days of the mother starting the pill. This does not occur in all mothers, but it certainly occurs in some. Even the progesterone only pill *sometimes* seems to cause a significant decrease. Whether it is true that it does cause fewer problems is difficult to prove, especially since it is used so much less often than combination oral contraceptives. It is also not a given that if the mother used the pill while nursing another baby without problems that there will be no problems with this particular baby. We have seen mothers with very dramatic

decreases in their milk supplies within 10 days of starting the very same pill at the very same time postpartum that they took with previous babies, where it caused no problem at all. We don't know at this point what factors seem to cause this decrease in some situations and not in others.

The approach here is to stop the birth control pill and to start the mother on domperidone, which will bring the milk supply back much more quickly than simply stopping the birth control pill. In fact, in many cases stopping the pill does not always bring back the supply. Metoclopramide (Reglan) may also be used, since it is rarely necessary for the mother to be on a galactogogue for more than a few weeks. Once the mother begins taking the medication, the milk supply usually rebounds very quickly, often within a few days. Domperidone, though not easily available in the USA, can be obtained at some compounding pharmacies with a physician's prescription. Further information about the use of domperidone can be found in chapter six.

2. **The mother is pregnant again.** Though it is rare for breastfeeding mothers, especially those *exclusively* breastfeeding, to become pregnant within the first 6 months, it does happen, and it happens more often once the baby is over 6 months of age. The hormones of pregnancy interfere with the effect of prolactin on the alveolar cells of the breast (just as the birth control pill does) and milk supply generally decreases.

If the baby is over 6 months of age and is eating other foods, there is usually no need to introduce formula and certainly no need to introduce a bottle. Introducing a bottle (even if the baby will take it, which is not guaranteed) when the mother's milk supply is down will very frequently lead to the baby's refusing the breast. Even if formula or other milk is desirable because of the drop in breastmilk production, there is no need for the baby to receive it in a bottle. The milk can be given by cup, mixed with solids, or given in the form of yogurt or cheese. There is no need for the baby to *drink* the milk. In some cases the baby will take the milk with a lactation aid, but this is not always easy with the older baby as they are more likely to notice and object to the tube's presence.

If the baby is under six months and not showing any signs of readiness for solids, then the mother can supplement with a lactation aid to avoid the baby refusing the breast. If the baby is under six months but over 4 months and seems willing to take solid foods, solids can be introduced instead of formula. Current recommendations are to breastfeed exclusively for six months, but if the baby is between four and six months and the options are to either introduce formula or solids, I believe that adding solids is often preferable and will help to maintain breastfeeding at the maximum level.

Though some believe that breastfeeding during pregnancy will increase the risk of spontaneous abortion, there is no evidence to support this. Many women (including Teresa, who breastfed through three of her four pregnancies) have breastfed through their pregnancies without difficulty.

3. **The mother is taking other drugs which decrease milk supply.** Several medications, without supportive data, are said to decrease milk supply. These include antihistamines which, based on our experience, should be used with caution in breastfeeding mothers. There have been occasions where mothers very definitely implicated them as a cause of decreased production. Since there are other medications that can be used to treat allergies (vasoconstrictive nose drops, steroid inhalers, antihistaminic eye drops, cromolyn, for example), it is possible in most cases to avoid antihistamine use by breastfeeding mothers. It should be remembered that antihistamines are also present in many "cold" medicines, so the mother may not be aware that this is what she has taken. Since most cold medicines are useless anyway, it would be better for breastfeeding mothers to avoid them altogether. Vasoconstrictive nose drops used with caution so as not to get rebound effects are a better choice for the nursing mother.

Diuretics, again without any good evidence, have been said to decrease milk supply as well. Although there is no proof, these too should be avoided by nursing mothers. Since there are a variety of other medications available for the treatment of hypertension and congestive heart failure, diuretics can almost always be avoided.

Recently, Hale has shown that a single dose of pseudoephedrine can decrease milk supply significantly. Interestingly, the more dramatic effects were in women whose milk supply was well established - the effect was more pronounced in mothers who had breastfed over 2 months. The decreased milk supply returned to pre-medication levels within 24 hours. However, the study looked only at the effect of a single 60 mg dose, and it cannot be said that return to pre-treatment levels would occur if the mother were on the medication for a week or two.

Two medications, bromocriptine and cabergoline, being antagonists of prolactin secretion are well known inhibitors of milk supply and should not be used for breastfeeding mothers.

4. **The mother is ill.** The most common cause of a decrease in milk supply due to illness in our experience is mastitis or a blocked duct. This is probably because the acute swelling of the breast compresses milk ducts around the affected area so the baby often finds it difficult to get milk from the breast. However, the decrease can also be persistent even once the mastitis or blocked duct has completely resolved. A decrease does not appear to be a usual result of either mastitis or blocked duct, but it does occur sometimes. Why the decrease should occur in some mothers and not in most is not clear. In our experience this does not appear related to the milk supply before the mastitis or blocked ducts, the type of treatment or lack of treatment for the mastitis or blocked duct, the number of previous episodes, or the age of the baby at the time of the problem. Treatment with domperidone does result in a full return of milk production in some cases, but definitely not all, though a partial return of milk supply does occur in the rest.

In addition to mastitis and blocked ducts, we have heard from many women that any type of febrile illness has been associated, in some instances, with a marked, sustained decrease in the milk supply. As in the case of blocked ducts and mastitis, this complication is not common, but it does occur. Domperidone helps in many cases, but it does not bring back the supply completely in every case.

5. **The mother has had an emotional "shock."** Every so often, we hear from a mother who has had an emotional trauma and says her milk "dried up." For example, they will tell us: "My mother died and the next day I had no more milk," or "My older child was admitted to the hospital and my milk disappeared." Fortunately, this reaction appears to be quite uncommon. Domperidone brings back the milk supply very rapidly and completely in such cases.

6. **The mother is feeding the baby on just one breast at each feeding.** Feeding on one breast at each feeding has become a common approach to dealing with some breastfeeding problems such as colic and slow weight gain (though the rationale for feeding a baby on just one side when the baby is not gaining well is a notion that I still cannot fathom). Since the milk increases in fat as the baby draws more out of the breast, the practice of "one breast per feeding" is based on the theory that longer feedings on one side will allow the baby to get more fat and thus more calories in the case of poor weight gain. Where this argument breaks down is that a baby is not getting milk simply because the baby is on the breast. If the baby is not getting any milk (often because of latch problems), the baby is obviously not getting high fat milk, so this approach to slow weight gain will be ineffective and could, in fact, make things worse. This approach sometimes works for "colic" when the mother has an abundant milk supply, but the end result is that the milk supply decreases. (Of course at times the goal is to reduce the milk supply in those cases where the mother's milk is overly-abundant.)

Instead, mothers should be advised to "finish" one side before offering the other. In some cases and at some feedings, this may mean that the baby doesn't take the second breast. Compression is a handy technique to help "finish" the first side before offering the other.

7. **There is more than occasional use of artificial nipples.** For various reasons, some mothers start to use bottles and pacifiers. This may be because they are going back to outside work, because they wish to stretch out the feedings, or to get the baby to sleep through the night. In any case, the stratagem often does not

work because the result is often a decrease in the milk supply, so the baby wants to feed more frequently. It is not possible in many cases of early return to outside work to do much about the need to use bottles (practically speaking, day care workers and baby sitters will not use cups for 2 month old babies), but there should be a determined effort to maintain the milk supply by frequent, effective pumping and effective breastfeeding when the mother is with the baby. In some cases it is possible for the baby to be brought to the mother's work or for the mother to go to the day care center to nurse. On-site day care is, of course, the best approach to a bad situation. A better approach would be a reasonable maternity leave (a minimum of 6 months, a year or more is better). Physicians should be in the forefront of lobbying for decent maternity leave.

In the case of the mother trying to stretch out the feedings or to get the baby to sleep through the night, counseling is often effective. *In our experience* mothers are willing to feed their babies more often, including during the night, when they understand why it is important, but they are often influenced by family, friends, and health professionals who tell them things like: "The baby is 3 months old and should be sleeping through the night. Your milk must not be rich enough, etc.."

I definitely see mothers whose babies abruptly slow down in their weight gain patterns after being "trained" to sleep all night. It is not true that the breasts will always compensate for the disappearance of night feedings by making more milk during the day. We know that women's breasts vary in their storage capacity and some women need those night feedings to be able to provide enough milk for their babies. Another thing I sometimes see is the baby who has learned to self-soothe at night starts doing it in the daytime, too. He's hungry, he looks around for mom and she's not right there, so he just sucks his thumb instead as he has learned to do to comfort himself at night. The result: he nurses less often and gets less and less milk. Mothers sometimes expect that if the baby is "truly hungry" he will cry and insist on being fed, but since the babies have learned that crying at night didn't bring anyone to come and feed them, they seem to believe that there is no point in crying to be fed during the day either.

Mothers who are considering trying "sleep training" programs should be made aware of the possible risks in terms of breastfeeding.

8. **The mother is trying to live up to society's unrealistic expectations.** Society expects, quite unrealistically, that once the baby is a few months old or even a few weeks old that taking care of the baby becomes a piece of cake and the mother is now expected to keep a tidy house, return to work outside the home, take care of aging parents, etc. Many mothers are doing too much. Not only are they taking care of a 3 or 4 month old, no easy task, but they are also driving older children to ballet or violin, handling shopping, household chores, volunteer work, etc. Having a new baby is nature's signal to slow down a bit. The dust bunnies under the bed can wait; there is no rush to get rid of them. There is nothing wrong with food being delivered from time to time (hint to grandparents—delivered home cooked meals are **always** better than fast food).

9. **Babies were scheduled or not fed very often in the early weeks.** This decrease in milk supply also happens with mothers who are scheduling or not feeding very often in the early weeks. You notice them when their babies are small because they will walk around with the baby, trying to entertain or distract him until they feel it is "time" to nurse. Sometimes they are following a program like Ezzo's "Growing Kids God's Way" with its "parent-directed feeding," but often they have just absorbed our cultural tendency to think babies shouldn't eat "too often." And because these mothers have an initially abundant milk supply, the babies gain weight well and the mother thinks everything is going fine. The mothers who do not have an abundant supply who are trying to feed this way usually end up changing how often they feed, supplementing, or giving up.

But we know from the research done on mothers who are pumping that frequency of pumping is more important than total amount of time spent pumping. In other words, mothers who pump for five minutes 6 times a day make more milk than mothers who pump for 10 minutes 3 times a day (as an example). Clearly this should apply to babies at the breast as well. So the mother who is nursing only 6 or 8 times a day will find, after the initial weeks of high production, that her milk supply starts to decrease. The baby starts to be frustrated and pull off, and the milk decreases still further.

The research on tribal societies has shown that babies there usually breastfeed very frequently – one study showed an average of 4 times an hour. Of course, there are also some mothers who do not feed according to the baby's need who continue to produce enough milk, but I think they are a minority.

This is not to say that mothers should be watching the clock and feeding every three hours instead of every four hours. It is about watching the baby's cues and putting him to the breast as soon as he shows interest rather than trying to put him off a little longer. The baby will not always go to the breast out of hunger. Maybe he is thirsty, tired and wanting to nurse to sleep, or something has startled him and he wants to nurse to be comforted.

In my experience, mothers who think about nurturing their babies at the breast rather than just feeding the baby at the breast, who will offer the breast any time the baby fusses or shows interest, rarely have difficulties with their milk supply dropping. Those frequent feedings, even if they are short, seem to do the trick.

10. **The baby's behavior changes with time.** Babies respond to milk flow. This is obvious to anyone who watches babies breastfeeding. It is the reason that the bottle interferes with breastfeeding, not only at the beginning of lactation, but even after milk supply is well established. In the first few weeks of life, a baby tends to fall asleep at the breast when the flow of milk is slow. But after the first 4 to 6 weeks, many babies tend to pull at the breast when the flow slows down. Of course, not all babies react in the same way. Some are pulling at the breast even from the first days; some always tend to fall asleep when the flow is slow regardless of their age; some may react differently depending on how hungry they are and how quickly the flow slows.

This is the scenario that we sometimes see: In the first few weeks after the initial rapid flow, the baby who does not have a very good latch may suck and sleep and suck without getting large quantities at this point. However, the mother will usually have more milk ejection reflexes and the baby will drink more - he has to, the milk will flow into his mouth without effort. When the mother's supply is abundant, the baby usually gains fine, though he may spend long periods on the breast *despite* the mother's abundant supply. However, as the baby gets older, the baby will start to pull away from the breast and usually the mother will then offer the other side. The same thing may happen on that breast. The baby pulls off the breast even though he has not "drained" the breast and even though he may still be a little hungry. If he is still a bit hungry, he may suck his hand rather than cry. Because of inefficient "draining" of the breast, the mother's milk supply decreases slightly. Over a few weeks, this may not make much difference especially if her milk production was very good to start with. But in some cases, eventually the supply decreases significantly, so the baby no longer gains well. He may even lose weight. Yet the mothers often describe the babies as being content and happy (as long as they suck their hand). The mothers often describe the baby's nursing as extremely rapid, often lasting no more than a couple of minutes before the baby pulls off the breast. In spite of the baby's obviously wishing to continue sucking, he will usually refuse to return to the breast unless the breast is "full." How the baby knows is a mystery, but there must be a distinctive aroma associated with the fuller or "empty" breast as the baby will refuse to continue on the breast he has just come off, fighting and crying even before latching on, but will immediately take the side where he has not yet nursed.

I believe this is the most common reason for late onset poor weight gain, in spite of good, or even better than good, weight gain for the first 2 to 3 months. I believe it is due to a poor latch in association with an abundant milk supply. The poorer the latch, the more the baby depends on the milk ejection reflex to get milk, and thus gets set up for poor weight gain after the first few weeks or months.

Our approach to this problem depends on increasing the milk supply. Though pumping can be helpful, it is not always practical for many mothers. We also find that if the problem has been going on for more than a few weeks, pumping alone rarely corrects the problem and certainly does not do so quickly. The same is true for more frequent feedings and even using compressions to get the baby to drink more. First, we teach the mother how to know a baby is getting milk at the breast (not just sucking) and then we instruct her to:

- Feed the baby on the first side, using compression when the milk intake by the baby slows down, squeezing the breast once the baby sucks but does not drink (see instruction sheet and video clips at www.breastfeedingonline.com).

- Switch sides when even compression does not seem to work or the baby pulls off the breast.

- Switch back and forth as long as the baby takes the breast and gets reasonable amounts of milk, but do not try to force the baby to continue breastfeeding if he resists.

- Use a lactation aid to supplement if it is urgent to get the baby gain weight (usually one can wait as in the case study). Our experience with babies such as this getting bottles for supplementation is that they quickly, within a couple of weeks *at the longest*, refuse to take the breast altogether.

- Start domperidone 30 mg three times a day.

- If the baby is older (5 or 6 months), start solids. It is still important to increase the breastmilk supply as well, so that the baby continues getting breastmilk and continues breastfeeding.

Continuation of JW's Case Study.

We suggested the above approach (not including supplementation or solids). One week after the initial visit, the baby weighed 5.92 kg (13 lb and a little less than half an ounce), but more important than this relatively small weight gain was that the mother felt she had more milk, stated that the baby drank longer at the breast, and noticed an increase in his urine output. Indeed, it was obvious on observation of a feeding that the baby was drinking better than the week before. Two weeks after the initial visit, the baby weighed 6.1 kg (13 lb 7 oz), and four weeks after the initial visit, 6.5 kg (14 lb 5 oz). At six months of age (about 2 months after the initial visit), he weighed 7.3 kg (16 lb 1 oz). The baby was still exclusively breastfed up to about 1 week before this last visit when the mother had started solids in response to the baby's obvious desire to start eating solids. Domperidone was weaned down over approximately 6 weeks time. The baby continued breastfeeding until he was 18 months of age.

This mother and baby's story is typical of what we see in our clinic at least 3 or 4 times a month. In most cases, there is no obvious reason for the milk supply to have decreased except this change in how the baby responds to decreased flow. Prevention would be simple: getting a good latch from the very first day, teaching mothers how to know the baby is getting milk (open mouth wide-->pause-->close mouth type of sucking), and "finishing" the first side before offering the second.

References

Righard L, Alade MO. Effect of delivery room routines on success of first breastfeed. *Lancet* 1990;336:1105-07.

Yamauchi Y, Yamanouchi I. The relationship between rooming in/not rooming and breastfeeding variables. *Acta Paediatr Scand* 1990;79:1017-22.

Yamauchi Y, Yamanouchi I. Breastfeeding frequency during the first 24 hours after birth in fullterm neonates. *Pediatrics* 1990;86:171-5.

Righard L, Alade MO. Sucking technique and its effect on success of breastfeeding. *Birth* 1992;19:185-9.

Cronenwett L, Stukel T, Kearney M, Barrett J, Covington C, Del Monte K, *et al*. Single daily bottle use in the early weeks postpartum and breastfeeding outcomes. *Pediatrics* 1992;90:760-6.

Nissen E, Lilja G, Matthiesen AS, Ransjo-Arvidsson AB, Uvnas-Moberg K, Widstrom AM. Effect of maternal pethidine on infants' developing breastfeeding behaviour. *Acta Paediatr* 1995;84:140-5.

Winberg J. Examining breastfeeding performance: forgotten influencing factors. *Acta Paediatr* 1995;84:465-7.

Wright A, Rice S, Wells S. Changing hospital practices to increase the duration of breastfeeding. *Pediatrics* 1996;5:669-75.

Saadeh R, Akre J. Ten steps to successful breastfeeding: a summary of the rationale and scientific evidence. *Birth* 1996;23:154-60.

Nissen E, Widstrom AM, Lilja G, Matthiesen AS, Uvnas-Moberg K, Jacobsson G, Boreus LO. Effects of routinely given pethidine during labour on infants' developing breastfeeding behaviour. Effects of dose—delivery time interval and various concentrations of pethidine/norpethidine in cord plasma. *Acta Paediatr* 1997;86:201-8.

Williams AF. Hypoglycaemia of the newborn: a review of the literature. *World Health Organization*, Geneva. 1997.

Kuan LW, Britto M, Decolongon J, Schoettker PJ, Atherton HD, Kotagal UR. Health system factors contributing to breastfeeding success. *Pediatrics* 1999;104;e28.

Riordan J, Gross A, Angeron J, Krumwiede B, Melin J. The effect of labor pain relief medication on neonatal suckling and breastfeeding duration. *J Hum Lact* 2000;16:7-12.

Hoseth E, Joergensen A, Ebbeson F, Moeller M. Blood glucose levels in a population of healthy breastfed, term infants of appropriate size for gestational age. *Arch Dis Child Fetal Neonatal Ed* 2000;83:F117-9.

Kramer MS, Chalmers B, Hodnett ED, Sevkovskaya Z, Dzikovich I, Shapiro S, *et al.* Promotion of breastfeeding intervention trial (PROBIT); a randomized trial in the republic of Belarus. *JAMA* 2001;285:413-20.

Varendi H, Porter RH. Breast odour as the onlymaternal stimulus elicits crawling towards the odour source. *Acta Paediatr* 2001;90:372-5.

Cattaneo A, Buzzetti R, on behalf of the Breastfeeding Research and Training Working Group. Effect on rates of breastfeeding on training for the Baby Friendly Hospital Initiative. *Br Med J* 2001;323:1358-62.

Newman J. Breastfeeding problems associated with early introduction of bottles and pacifiers. *J Hum Lact* 1990;6:59-63.

Lang S, Lawrence CJ, L'E Orme, R. Cup feeding: an alternative method of infant feeding. *Arch Dis Child* 1994;71:365-9.

Armstrong H. Techniques of feeding infants: the Case for Cup Feeding. *Research in Action* 1998;no 8:1-6.

Howard CR, de Blieck EA, ten Hoopen CB, Howard FM, Lanphear BP, Lawrence RA. Physiologic stability of newborns during cup and bottle feeding. *Pediatrics* 1999;104:1204-7.

Malhotra N, Vishwambaran L, Sundaram KR, Narayanan I. A controlled trial of alternative methods of oral feeding in neonates. *Early Hum Dev* 1999;54:29-38.

Gupta A, Khanna K, Chattree S. Cup feeding: an alternative to bottle feeding in a neonatal intensive care unit. *J Trop Pediatr* 1999;45:108-110.

Aljazak K, Hale TW, Ilett KF, Hartmann PE, Mitoulas LR, Kristensen JH, Hackett LP. 2003. Pseudophedrine: effects on milk production in women and estimation of infant exposure via breastmilk. *Br J Clin Pharmacol.* Jul:56(1):18-24.

The Baby Who Refuses to Eat

A common problem pediatricians face and we face at our breastfeeding clinic is the toddler (for example, a child around 14 months old) who only breastfeeds and refuses to eat other foods. Too often, the parents receive the advice that they must wean the child from breastfeeding so that he or she will eat. While this approach may works sometimes, it is not the only one and certainly not the best approach. For one thing, forcing a 9 month old, 14 month old, or 21 month old to wean who does not want to wean can be a devilish enterprise that can exhaust the parents and cause great distress to and feelings of rejection in the child.

Prevention

Just as the breastfed baby should be fed when the baby desires to be fed, there is no reason to add solids in a rigid way with prescribed amounts of certain foods which must be consumed by a certain age. With younger babies, we have the problem of feeding by the clock; with older babies, the problem becomes feeding according to the calendar. Neither is appropriate.

Now that most professional societies are urging exclusive breastfeeding until 6 months or so, it should be noted that many babies of this age will not eat the processed infant cereals which have been the "mainstay" of first solids in western countries for a long time. The cereals do not taste particularly good and many babies of this age will refuse it, not always after one feeding of it, but some will spit it out the first time they taste it. I believe it is time to rethink the whole notion of "cereal as first food" because our insistence on it may directly lead to feeding problems. It does not take many feedings of cereal for the child to understand that this is not good stuff that's coming towards his face. Instead of letting it into his mouth and spitting it out, he will turn his head away and we now have a "feeding problem."

I believe a much less rigid approach to starting solids will prevent the majority of food refusal problems. Babies naturally want to eat food. They show this from fairly early on. By 4 months of age, many babies sitting on their mother's or father's lap while the parent is eating will become very interested in what's going on in the plate, what's happening with this fork moving from plate to mouth, and what are these chewing movements of the parent's mouth. They will watch the fork move back and forth from plate to mouth and back to plate again. They are obviously fascinated. By the time they are 5 to 6 months of age, they start to try to grab at the fork or the food in the plate and try to put the food into their mouths. It seems to me that the baby has shown he is ready to eat. Does it matter if he is only 5 months and 3 weeks of age? Does it really matter that the general recommendation is that the baby does not need solids until 6 months of age? That is a general recommendation for the world, not every individual. It is true that the baby does not usually "need" food until about 6 months or even later, but that does not mean the parents should be advised never to give food until 6 months.

And if the food the baby wants to eat happens to be mashed potatoes and not cereal, should we take the mashed potatoes out of his hand, slap his wrist, and give him cereal instead? I think this is not respecting the child as an individual, as someone who is part of the family. "No, even though you are obviously ready for our food, you get cereal." It should be noted that a generation ago, many physicians were suggesting cereal by the time the baby was a month or 6 weeks of age. By the time they were 6 months of age, they were eating everything: meat, vegetables, fruit. To say that if the baby starts eating solids at 6 months, he must start with processed cereals and go through the routine of one food a week, only a tablespoon or two at most twice a day, and all the rest of the rules makes no sense.

I have heard the argument that a baby of six months or so will put anything into his mouth, even that which is not food. Exactly. Good. Then you gently take the rubber band or the stone out of his hand and tell him by doing so, not necessarily in words, that that's not food. That's how he learns what food is. Putting the rubber band or the stone into his mouth and trying to eat them is the way he figures out what is and what isn't food. Of course if he is breastfeeding, the exposure to all sorts of bacteria on the rubber band and stone in the presence of breastfeeding helps him develop immunity to those bacteria. If you take the piece of pasta out of his hand and give him cereal, you tell him pasta is not food. If you take the strip of steak away from him, you tell him that's not food either.

I have heard the old saw about the necessity of giving one food at a time, so that if the baby is allergic to it, the parents will know. Really, how will they know? It is amazing what parents interpret as "allergy." A rash, true, can be an allergic response, but babies get rashes all the time, most of which probably have nothing to do with allergy. Parents often interpret vomiting and/or diarrhea after eating a food as allergy or "sensitivity" to that food when in fact these probably have nothing to do with sensitivity, at least most of the time. Vomiting is often due to the baby's not liking the food. Diarrhea may be completely unrelated to allergy.

A 9 month old grabs a piece of tomato and puts it into his mouth. Later, we see the skin around his lips is all red. The first reaction of many parents is: "He's allergic to tomato." Actually not, since it is the acid in the tomato juice which has caused the redness, but he will be labeled "allergic" and may never eat tomato again, poor child.

The fact of the matter is that if a baby starts eating food at 5 or 6 or 7 months of age or older, he can eat almost anything (though one would not want to give him round foods that can easily slip into the trachea - peanuts come immediately to mind). There is no need to go one food at a time, and there is no need to limit quantities. The baby should eat what and how much he wants. Then eating is pleasurable, and the baby is now part of the family in this very important way. Of course the breast is still providing most of his nutrition, but he is eating just like a "big person" with regard to solids.

What about the issue of babies' needing cereals in order to get iron? Actually, the iron in cereal is relatively poorly absorbed, with perhaps only 5% of the iron in cereal being absorbed into the baby's system. Furthermore, some cereals are quite constipating, particularly those made with rice. Whether it is the rice or the iron or both that causes the babies to be constipated is uncertain, since everyone denies the possibility of the cereals causing constipation. Mothers know better. I hear from many mothers whose babies never had anything like constipation until they started cereal. The mothers tend to keep on feeding those cereals, though, because they are convinced by their doctors that the baby needs them to get enough iron. Actually, many foods can give the baby iron. Meat is a good example. So is fish. The iron from both these foods is better absorbed by far than the iron from cereal. And if the baby is starting solids at 5 to 6 months of age, there is no reason that they cannot eat meat.

This approach, I believe, would prevent the majority of problems of babies eating solids that we see.

The child of 6 months or over who refuses food

There are two types of babies that fall into this category. The ones who are gaining weight well, and those who are not.

In the first case, the baby who is gaining weight well will usually eventually start eating well. Sometimes, he does not start eating until he is a year or more, but interestingly, though pediatricians often worry about iron deficiency anemia and zinc deficiency, our experience is that the child only occasionally becomes deficient in either iron or zinc. It would be wrong to say never, but it is interesting because in the cases when the child is not deficient the math just doesn't work. In our pediatric training, we had it all worked out. If the child is born at term and there is no unusual bleeding, he has iron stores in his body that will last him 4 to 6 months if he is breastfeeding exclusively, given the amount of iron he is born with and the amount he absorbs from breastmilk. However, one study has shown that babies can be exclusively breastfed to 9 months and only about 15% become iron deficient and almost none become anemic. The worry about poor development due to iron deficiency is with regard to anemia, not iron deficiency strictly speaking. You are iron deficient before you become anemic. Furthermore, more and more researchers are questioning what normal levels of iron are for the 6 month old child. What can be said of this question of iron is that we really don't know. I have seen a 14 month old, exclusively breastfeeding, no solid foods, no vitamins or supplements, no anything else, who had perfectly normal iron levels in his blood and no evidence of anemia. The math just doesn't work. He eventually started eating the next month. However, if there is real concern, the baby can be given medicinal iron and/or zinc in liquid form until he is ready to eat. Forcing such a baby, indeed *any* baby, to eat food is usually a lost cause.

But what about the baby who is not gaining, even losing weight? This is a different situation completely. I have already discussed reasons why a mother's milk might decrease in another chapter. In the situation discussed there, the baby pulls away from the breast and sucks his hand after a very short period of time on the breast. This baby almost always will accept food very easily, and the question of not eating does not arise. Of course, I believe that the mother should increase her milk supply, and if efforts to do so are not working, then domperidone should be used to increase the milk supply. Food will help the baby gain weight better, but breastmilk and breastfeeding are more than food, and we should make efforts to get the breastfeeding working better as well.

However, in some cases, when the milk supply decreases, the baby may react differently from the baby mentioned above. Instead of pulling away from the breast when the flow of milk slows, the baby will actually continue to suck at the breast for long periods of time. Sometimes such babies are on the breast for very long periods of time, most of the day in fact, or they have a pacifier in their mouths for long periods as well. In this case, the baby substitutes sucking at the breast for food. Sucking at the breast is pleasurable for the baby as it results in oxytocin release which gives him pleasurable feelings. Normally, one would expect him to accept food readily, and some will, but many do not. Why won't he accept food when he is not gaining weight, or in rare occasions, even losing weight? I have to admit I don't have an answer for this. But I do think I have an approach that does not include forced weaning of the baby from the breast.

If you watch a baby at the breast, you can tell when he is actually drinking milk and when he is not. This has been discussed elsewhere and can be seen on video at the websites www.thebirthden.com/Newman. html, www.breastfeedingonline.com, www.gentlemothering.ca, and other websites as well. In addition, the pause in the chin that shows the baby is getting milk can be seen on the instructional DVD on breastfeeding, *Dr. Jack Newman's Visual Guide to Breastfeeding.* When you watch the baby in the situation above (on the breast for long periods, refusing food, not gaining weight), you will see that he spends an inordinate amount of time "nibbling" on the breast, or put another way, very little time actually drinking at the breast. Thus, what many health professionals tell mothers, that the baby is filling up on breastmilk and that's why the baby is refusing to eat, just isn't true. It does not even make sense. If the baby were truly "filling up," the baby would be gaining weight well. I believe that this observation is at least partly responsible for many health professionals' telling parents that there is no nutritional value to breastmilk after 6 months or a year. The simple observation of a feeding and being able to distinguish when the baby is getting milk and when he is not can help dispel these strange notions. Instead of telling mothers they must forcibly wean the baby, the knowledge of what is going on while the baby is breastfeeding can help us find an approach that is more breastfeeding friendly.

First of all, the mother needs to know when the baby is getting milk and when the baby is not. This is easily taught once the health practitioner knows how. In fact, I think this technique should be routinely taught to mothers during the first days after the baby's birth (yes indeed, you can see that pause even on day one, though it is not as obvious). Then the mother can follow the Protocol to Increase Breastmilk Intake by the Baby. She feeds the baby on one side until the baby does not drink any more, then uses compression while he is nibbling to increase his intake of breastmilk (yes, we want to increase the baby's intake of breastmilk not decrease it). The use of compression can be helpful here, but if the milk supply has been down for quite some time, it may take time for the milk supply to increase, even somewhat. This is true for pumping as well. Though I wouldn't completely condemn the idea, to tell you the truth, I am not keen on pumping in this situation for the following reasons:

1. Pumping is expensive (to rent or buy the machine).

2. Pumping is tiring and time consuming, and in this situation, when will the mother do the pumping? Between breastfeeds? In the cases discussed in this chapter, there is almost no "between breastfeeds."

3. Pumping diminishes the mother's enjoyment of breastfeeding.

4. Pumping, if not done properly, can cause sore nipples.

5. In spite of everything we tell mothers about not being able to tell how much you are producing or can produce, mothers look at what they pump and get discouraged.

6. Compression is like pumping, but instead of pumping into a bottle, the mother expresses into the baby.

However, as with compression, pumping may take a long time to really start making a difference. Thus, I will often prescribe domperidone to the mother in this situation. It may require the emphasis of repetition, but yes, I believe the best approach is not stopping breastfeeding, but rather increasing the intake of breastmilk by the baby.

Once the mother has fed the baby on both sides and the baby no longer drinks, she then takes the baby off the breast and offers food. Not forces, but offers food, perhaps tasting some herself to show that she enjoys eating (a good reason to not offer cereal or other processed baby foods if you have to taste it yourself). If there are older siblings, it is often a good idea to have them try to feed the baby. Babies, even those younger than 9 months of age, recognize that these are children, are fascinated by them, and often copy what they do. If there are no older children in the family, the mother may go to a parent drop in center around lunch time or snack time, and the baby seeing others eat may be convinced that this is a good idea. Again, forcing is not a good idea. Indeed, an 8 or 9 month old baby is very keen to demonstrate his competence and independence. All parents are aware that the 8 or 9 month old may not accept a spoon full of food and will instead try to grab the spoon out of the parent's hand and try to feed himself, even if he does turn the spoon upside down as it approaches his mouth.

If necessary iron and, if useful, zinc can be given by eyedropper into the corner of the baby's mouth while the baby is on the breast, as they will accept these medicines better this way than trying to force them to take them after the feeding. It was thought that these babies would not eat because they were zinc deficient. Zinc deficiency is associated with loss of appetite, but our experience has not shown that they eat better simply by giving them zinc.

Once these babies start getting more food, they tend to start eating more – that's the nice circle, rather than the vicious circle. In some parts of Africa that I visited, these babies would often be admitted to the hospital, a tube put into their stomachs and they would be given nourishment in this way, and usually once their deficiencies were made up and they started to gain weight, they would start to eat. Notice that breastfeeding was *never* stopped, at least in those places I visited. I would not agree with this approach especially in more affluent countries because there is no rush to get the baby eating. If he has not gained weight for 2 months, do we have to turn everything around tomorrow? If the baby is losing weight, the situation is more delicate. Sometimes hospitalization can help, the baby may start to eat more when others feed him solids. This is not to suggest that the parents are not competent, but rather that babies react differently to different people.

In summary, the situation of the older baby only staying on the breast and not gaining weight can be prevented by making sure the mother does not get a late onset decrease in her milk supply (see previous chapter). I believe this decrease in milk supply between 2 and 5 months of age is the primary cause of the problem, with the baby staying on the breast for long periods of time and substituting sucking at the breast for eating food. Ultimately, the prevention of the problem goes back to the first days when we should be teaching mothers how to breastfeed properly which, unfortunately, is not the case in too many hospitals across the world.

The second aspect of preventing this problem is to follow the baby's cues when the baby is ready to eat and not depend on the calendar, schedules, or meal plans for toddlers. Long ago, in the 1920's, it was shown that given the choice of a wide variety of foods, babies would eat what they need in amounts that they need.

Finally, this problem can be usually fixed without stopping breastfeeding. Forced weaning in any situation is not a good idea. In the case of poor weight gain in the toddler, it is even a less good idea. I am reminded of a 15 month old child who was "breastfeeding only" (in quotes because she was probably not breastfeeding much), who would eat only jello, and maintained her weight but did not gain. The mother was convinced to wean her. The child not only did not start to eat, but now did not have breastmilk either. Instead of maintaining her weight, she actually started to lose. Resolving this problem then became a long and difficult process.

12 Case Studies

These are cases Teresa has encountered with comments from Jack in parentheses within each study and further comments from Teresa at the end of each description. One point we hope you will recognize from these cases is that you don't have to be a doctor (or nurse) to help mothers with most of these issues. Also, in some cases, Jack would have made somewhat different recommendations than Teresa did – but that doesn't mean Teresa's approach was wrong. There is usually more than one way to solve a problem, and often it takes some trial and error to figure out what will work best in any given situation.

A baby who wouldn't latch

When I first saw this mother, the baby was three weeks old. The mother had gone into labor normally but as soon as she arrived at the hospital, the baby was determined to be in a breech position and an emergency C-section was done. The baby was very quiet and sleepy after the birth. Although he was eventually brought to her when he was about two hours old, he showed no interest in nursing. **(This is two hours too late. There is no reason a baby who is well, as this baby was after a cesarean section, should be separated from his mother. See the photo of a baby skin-to-skin with his mother while they are still sewing her up after a cesarean section.)** He was brought to her for feedings at regular intervals after that, but continued to be uninterested and unwilling to take the breast **(Babies need to be with their mothers, skin-to-skin. As Dr. Nils Bergmann says, the baby's normal habitat is the mother, skin-to-skin. Had this baby been with the mother, she could have picked up feeding cues that would have avoided "no feeding" for 12 hours.)**

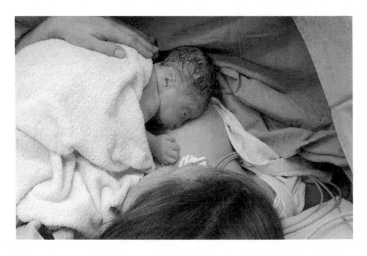

When he was 12 hours old, the nursing staff began to be more concerned that he had not fed. **(Why were the staff concerned? What evidence do we have that 12 hours is too long for a baby on the first day of life not to feed. We know that babies born without any medication after a normal birth do exactly as this baby did.)** After repeated and increasingly forceful attempts to get him to feed **(Forcing the baby to the breast is exactly the way to ensure the baby will develop an aversion to the breast)**, she was advised to pump her milk and finger-feed him. This is how he was fed over the next few days. **(Finger feeding is not primarily a method to avoid bottles, but rather an approach to get the baby to take the breast. Finger feeding should be used to calm the baby, get the baby sucking well, and once this has occurred - and this takes only about 30 to 60 seconds of finger feeding - the baby can be moved to the breast.)** By the time he was a week old, she had decided that the finger-feeding was too slow and was giving him her milk in a bottle. **(Finger feeding can be slow, but the point is that finger feeding is not primarily a way of feeding the baby, but rather a way of preparing the baby to take the breast. But in the first few days, when the baby does not need a lot, it can be used to feed the baby, if necessary.)** She made occasional attempts to offer the breast, but found he would immediately cry and turn away when held in the cross-cradle position.

The mother had plenty of milk and was easily able to pump enough for him, but was finding it very time-consuming.

When I saw the mother and baby, we first gave him an ounce of milk from the bottle so that he wouldn't be too hungry, then tried to feed him in the cross-cradle position. **(A baby who is ravenous will likely not take the breast. If he's angry enough he may not even take a bottle.)** As soon as his mother held him on her arm and against her body, he began to cry and struggle. When she went to cuddle him against her shoulder, he put his hands to his mouth and showed all the signs of being hungry, but moving him back into a feeding position led to more crying, pushing away, and flailing around.

Since the baby reacted so strongly to being held in the cross-cradle position, I thought it might work to try something different, so we used the football hold. He didn't seem to associate this with being forced onto the breast and was much more relaxed. We took things slowly and carefully with the goal of keeping him calm. His mother kept her hand behind his neck and shoulder, not touching his head at all, aimed her nipple at his nose, and brushed his top lip with her breast below the nipple. His mouth seemed to open automatically, he immediately latched on and fed beautifully. He was obviously swallowing milk and looked relaxed and blissful.

After that one feeding, this little guy never looked back. His mother fed him using the football hold for the next few days and then decided to switch over to the cross-cradle and cradle holds. She called me at that point because her nipples were getting sore. I was able to help her improve her latch technique in the cross-cradle position, to get a deeper and more asymmetric latch, and she found it much more comfortable.

(By using the cross cradle hold and asking the mother to compress the breast as the baby comes onto the breast so he gets a gush of milk, the same thing can be accomplished.)

Comments on this case: I see many babies who have become completely aversive to even being held in a breastfeeding position because of repeated attempts to force them to take the breast. Using a different position sometimes helps; some babies need to have some relaxed time "hanging out at the breast" before they will feel comfortable enough to attempt breastfeeding. It sometimes works to have the mother sit in a warm bath with the baby – the warm water seems to relax everybody. She can let the baby lie on her chest while she leans back against the end of the tub. Often the baby will begin to seek out the breast on his own, just as babies do right after birth. Also, notice that getting a good latch in one position (in this case, the football hold) doesn't guarantee that mother and baby will automatically get a good latch in a different position.

Another non-latching baby

I saw this mother and baby at a much earlier stage – 24 hours after birth. The baby, a girl, was born at home after a normal and uneventful birth, but had either slept or looked quietly around her since then. She'd shown no interest in breastfeeding at all, and the mother's and midwife's gentle attempts to encourage her had no effect.

When I tried to latch the baby, she simply didn't open her mouth. Even when I stroked her lip with my finger, she clamped her mouth closed and refused to open it. This wasn't the angry response of the very aversive baby, but we still weren't getting any milk into her.

I showed the mother how to hand-express her milk and suggested that she could feed the baby small amounts of colostrum using a syringe or try giving her some from a spoon. I also encouraged her to keep the baby skin-to-skin continuously for the next day or two.

She called me the next morning to say that she had been lying on her back in bed with the baby sleeping on her abdomen, skin-to-skin. The baby woke up from her nap and began to crawl towards the breast. Within minutes, she latched on and nursed effectively and enthusiastically for almost half an hour. After a short break (and the passing of some meconium), the mother helped the baby to the second breast and found that she readily and eagerly latched on. From this point on, the baby breastfed beautifully.

Comments on this case: Why did this baby not breastfeed for the first 36 hours? I don't know. I do know that when my first son was born nearly 30 years ago, the normal hospital routine was to not allow babies to breastfeed for the first 24 hours. So in those days, this baby would have been one of the few that was happy with that routine! Now most hospitals will insist on supplementation, usually with formula, if the baby has not breastfed within 12 hours. I think this case also demonstrates the importance of skin-to-skin contact. For many of these reluctant nursers, spending time skin-to-skin with their mothers seems to "wake up" the baby's breastfeeding instincts. **(It also demonstrates that it may be normal for some babies not to be interested in breastfeeding for 24 hours and often much longer. In fact early on at the breastfeeding clinic, I came across a mother who had both children at home, and insisted they did not seem the least bit interested in breastfeeding for 5 full days, and then just started as if they had been doing it all their lives. Neither baby got sick, neither baby got dehydrated, obviously neither baby had received any medication during the labor. The 3 year old was with the mother and the 3 month old and obviously both were quite normal. I think we have a problem because we don't know what normal is. Of course, with the use of medications during labor, the situation is further complicated. I can honestly say too, that I would never have been as calm as this mother seems to have been about the babies not feeding at all for the first five days. When would I have gotten nervous? Certainly by 3 days, but when? I don't think I can put a number on it.)**

Latch or inadequate breast tissue?

This baby girl weighed nearly ten pounds at birth, but when I saw her at two weeks, she had still not regained her birthweight. The mother had been told by the hospital staff that she probably had inadequate breast tissue as her breasts were widely spaced and somewhat tubular in shape. (I have now seen a few women who have these types of breasts and manage to breastfeed just fine. In two cases, weight gain was slow for the first few weeks, but then the babies took off. In another case, the mother came to me prenatally because she wanted to make sure she wouldn't have any problems and we worked in the same pediatric unit. I was discouraged to see her extremely "tubular" breasts, but did not say anything except my usual prenatal advice. She never had the slightest problem with breastfeeding or milk supply. We should be careful of this "inadequate breast tissue" diagnosis.) She had noticed only minor changes in her breasts during the pregnancy (her first). **(The first woman who came to our clinic with what I realized was an "overabundance" of milk claimed to have no breast changes during the pregnancy. After the first pregnancy, obvious breast changes do not always**

occur.) Test weighings showed that the baby was only getting about an ounce at each feeding, and the mother had begun to supplement with formula. **(I must say that I am very much against test weighings. We do not have an idea of how much a baby is supposed to get at any given time. We cannot say that if a baby is "supposed" to get x amount of formula because of such and such a weight, that this also applies to breastmilk. I think that test weighings do nothing but cause anxiety for the mother and the staff.)** The mother also complained of very sore nipples. **(This means the baby was not latching on well.)**

I reassured the mother that even if she wasn't able to produce a full milk supply, getting a good latch would ensure that the baby got the maximum amount of milk. So we would work first on improving the latch.

When I watched the baby at the breast, the latch was not ideal. In part, I think, because of the shape of the mother's breasts. The baby seemed to have some difficulty in getting her chin well into the breast, and I needed to gently press on her bottom lip to help it flange outward. When we made these small adjustments to get a more asymmetrical latch and used some breast compression as well, the baby did begin swallowing milk, but the mother was still experiencing considerable pain. When the baby let go, the mother's nipple was shaped like a new lipstick with a line of blisters along the edge. A quick check of the baby's mouth and tongue showed that she had a significant tongue-tie – the end of the tongue was clearly heart-shaped and its motion restricted by the tight frenulum.

We were able to arrange to have the frenulum clipped the next day, and the mother noticed an immediate improvement – feedings were much less painful. However, the baby continued to need adjustment each time she latched on to ensure that her mouth was open wide enough and her bottom lip flanged out. It became part of the mother's nursing routine – latch the baby on, then use a finger to press gently on the chin and flip the bottom lip out – and the baby was quite accepting. The mother was able to stop the formula supplements within a day or two and continue exclusively breastfeeding. This baby was a fairly slow-gaining baby throughout her first year, but it was a slow and steady gain and she was healthy and energetic.

Comments on this case: I think this example is a good reminder that we need to consider all the possible factors when there is a problem. My first reaction in looking at this mother's unusually-shaped breasts was that she would not be able to breastfeed exclusively, as the hospital staff had said. However, the real problem in this baby's lack of weight gain was a poor latch complicated still further by tongue-tie. Once those were dealt with, the baby was able to get all the milk she needed. Even when other factors seem to be present, getting the best latch possible allowed the baby to get all the available milk.

Six months of painful feedings

This baby girl was nearly six months old when I first saw her, but she had been seen by many others prior to this. The mother described what she felt during feedings as "toe-curling, heel-slamming pain." She'd had this intense pain from the very first time her baby went to the breast and had been told that this was normal and would disappear as her nipples toughened up. It did not go away. Her nipples were scabbed, bleeding and raw on the ends.

The mother had a very strong commitment to breastfeeding, and could see that her daughter was thriving, gaining well, and enjoying breastfeeding. So she persisted, despite the pain. She saw several public health nurses as well as her family doctor who all felt the latch looked good and could not explain her ongoing, constant pain.

When I finally met this mother and baby, I made a huge mistake. I assumed that because of the number of people she had seen, by something as basic as tongue-tie would have been ruled out. It was only at our second meeting when I sat watching her baby play on her lap that I realized the baby never stuck her tongue out. I asked to check the baby's tongue and, sure enough, the frenulum was very tight and significantly restricting the motion of the tongue.

Even after the frenulum was clipped (by Dr. Newman), the mother continued to experience some pain. She went back to see Dr. Newman, and he recognized that the many months of trauma to her nipples had set up a perfect environment for yeast. After two weeks of treatment for the yeast infection, the mother told me she picked up her baby one day to nurse and realized – "it didn't hurt. It was pure bliss. It was everything I'd dreamed of."

Comments on this case: First, this mother's determination to continue breastfeeding and to keep looking for help with her difficulties even when the first people she sought out weren't able to solve the problems is impressive. I find this case is an important reminder to me not to assume that the people who had seen the mother previously would have covered all the "basics." Ask the questions, watch the baby feed, check the tongue and palate, no matter what. It only takes a few minutes and helps ensure something crucial won't be missed. Finally, this case also shows how nipple damage due to latch problems (related to tongue-tie in this situation, but other latch problems also cause nipple damage) can create the perfect setting for yeast or bacterial infections in the nipple and breast, so we should be watching for these even as we improve the latch.

Mother with very large breasts

This baby was about four days old when I first saw him and was being primarily bottlefed with occasional attempts at the breast because the mother was having such difficulty in latching him. Her breasts were large and soft. She was concerned because she had not noticed the feeling of engorgement that everyone told her she would feel; even at four days her breasts were definitely not firm or engorged.

When she tried to feed the baby in the cross-cradle hold, it was almost comical. She positioned the baby on her arm, undid her nursing bra, and the baby disappeared under her breast. When she used one hand to support her breast, she could not find a comfortable position that allowed her to get the baby latched on.

I suggested that we try lying down as I've found this position useful for other women with very large breasts. Using pillows to support the mother in a stable and comfortable position lying on her side, we then arranged the baby. His body formed a letter V with the mother's body. His feet and legs were against her stomach, his head was at the bottom of her breast, and the nipple was pointed at his nose. The mother put her hand behind his back at the base of his neck and brought him in close to the breast. I had to let her know when he was opening his mouth wide as she couldn't see it, but after a couple of times she was able to feel the movement of his bottom lip and jaw against the bottom of her breast and recognize this as the sign to help him complete the latch by tucking him in close to her.

For the first few weeks, this mother fed the baby lying down every time. She never did feel engorged, her breasts continued to feel soft, but the baby was gaining well. When she wanted to try feeding him sitting up, we experimented with positions and found that it worked well to have the mother sit cross-legged with her back against a straight surface (such as the wall behind her bed). The baby lay against her leg with his head on her knee. This put him level with her nipple. She used one hand to support her breast so the nipple was aimed at the baby's nose. The other hand behind the baby's back kept him on his side and turned towards her and moved him onto the breast when he opened his mouth wide to latch. While this position would not have worked for many women, it worked beautifully for this mother and her baby.

Comments on this case: The principles of a good latch are always the same, but sometimes you need to get a little creative in order to achieve it! I have noticed other large-breasted women not experiencing any engorgement (or very little), but this does not seem to affect their milk production.

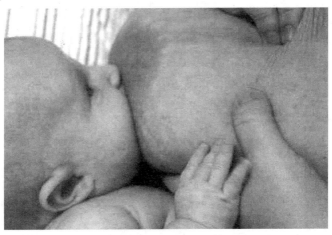

Mother with very large breasts (not the case discussed above). It took the mother 1 month to get the baby to latch on without our help. The problem was essentially a mechanical one of not being able to manipulate the breasts and the baby, not "flat nipples," "baby's small mouth," and all the usual reasons.

Baby with cranio-facial deformities

This baby girl was born with an unusual facial structure and webbed hands and feet. The physicians who saw her initially believed that she would also be developmentally delayed, but this was later shown to be an error. (The baby did not have the syndrome the doctors originally diagnosed). Her mother was told that breastfeeding would be impossible and not to bother trying.

I first saw this mother when her daughter was three days old. Despite the dire predictions, the mother very much wanted to breastfeed. My initial concern was that with the other deformities, the baby might have a cleft palate or unusually high palate. However, when we looked at her mouth everything seemed normal and the baby was able to suck well on my finger. She had a very receding chin and less flexibility in her jaw than most babies, but it certainly seemed worthwhile to try breastfeeding. After some trial and error, we found that the football hold seemed to work best. In that position, the weight of the mother's breast seemed to push against the receding chin and help her mouth stay open wide. The baby nursed well and looked relaxed and satisfied when she let go.

With continued support, this baby breastfed until she was two and a half years old. At that point she had facial surgery to correct some of the bone deformities that were causing her health problems and pain. She didn't go back to the breast afterwards.

Comments on this case: You never know until you try! Over the years I've seen a number of babies born with deformities, health problems and syndromes, and the majority of these mothers are told that their babies won't be able to breastfeed. Sometimes that is true, **(but only true possibly because we didn't try until much later than we should have)** although it may simply be that I don't have the skill and expertise to make breastfeeding work for that mother and baby. But in many cases, breastfeeding is possible. Sometimes the mother needs to use an unusual position, at least initially, to compensate for the baby's particular challenges. The key to making it work is keeping in mind what the latch needs to achieve – the nipple at the back of the baby's mouth, the lower jaw covering more of the breast than the upper jaw, the tongue forward and cupping the breast. Then you do whatever you need to do to make that happen. With Trisomy (and some other conditions), the large tongue may make latching difficult, but often allowing the baby's head to tip well back encourages the tongue to drop to the bottom of the baby's mouth and opens the throat wide so the milk flows right in and is not blocked by the tongue. It is always worth a try. Even if the baby gets little milk at the breast and needs supplementation, the baby benefits from breastfeeding.

Premature baby

This baby boy was born at 32 weeks weighing 3 pounds 12 ounces. **(A baby of 32 weeks can start Kangaroo Mother Care and can go to the breast immediately when he is stable.)** He was gavage fed for the first two and a half weeks with the mother's pumped milk. At that time she was told she could try him with a bottle for two feedings each day. **(There is no reason to start with bottles. Bottles interfere with breastfeeding and are not less stressful for the baby than the breast, on the contrary.)** When he had taken the bottle well for a couple of days, she was told to try feeding him at the breast twice a day using a nipple shield. **(And why the nipple shield????)** The baby was also given a pacifier between feedings. **(Instead of Kangaroo Mother Care and access to the breast)** The mother gradually worked up to six feedings at the breast each day with the nipple shield and two with the bottle. At this point the baby was five weeks old and was discharged from the hospital.

The mother contacted me four days later because she disliked using the nipple shield, bottles, and pacifiers and simply wanted to breastfeed. **(The normal response of a mother to all these unnecessary gadgets!)** Her nipples were fairly small and flat, and when she attempted to put the baby to the breast without the shield, the baby did not respond at all – he would open his mouth but not suck. She had some nipple damage and felt that with the shield on, the baby was compressing her nipple with his gums.

The first step we took was to eliminate the pacifier and move away from the scheduled, every three hour feedings that had been instituted in the hospital. I tried to help the mother recognize the baby's feeding cues and see them as signals to offer the breast rather than to give a pacifier. Since the baby was still small and would easily shut down if he was frustrated, we had to take things slowly and try different approaches to see what he would tolerate. Weaning him from the shield and bottles was a slow process that took more than a month. What seemed to work best was to start him off on the shield, then when he came to a natural pause in his feeding, remove the shield and offer him the nipple without it. But this did not work every time, and often he would cry and turn away from the breast without the shield. We tried a lactation aid at the breast but that seemed to also upset him. With the bottle feedings, we tried giving him a small amount from the bottle first, then offering the breast. Again, this worked sometimes but not always. The mother continued to pump three times a day to help maintain her milk supply and this milk was given in the bottle (or the lactation aid when we were trying that).

This mother needed a lot of support and encouragement through this process as she often felt that her baby was rejecting her breast and preferred the bottle and the nipple shield. Feedings were not relaxing and enjoyable at this point, but complicated and often frustrating. However, she was eventually able to exclusively breastfeed her baby without the shield or bottles, and stopped pumping as well. At this point her baby's rate of weight gain also improved – in fact, he became one of those big, chubby "blue-ribbon" babies despite being a slow starter. **(This whole problem could have been avoided if the special care unit did not stick to "traditional" approaches to breastfeeding the premature baby. With early Kangaroo Mother Care, avoidance of bottles and pacifiers, and feeding the baby according to cue, this baby could have been breastfed very soon after birth.)**

Comments on this case: I wanted to share this story because I see so many premature babies who have been through this same (or a similar) regimen: scheduled feedings, bottles introduced before the breast, nipple shields, and pacifiers. I've heard the rationale for it **(there is no rationale for it, it's just what we've always done—the evidence for use of nipple shields and bottles is not strong, and experience in other parts of the world show very well that in most cases they are not necessary)**, but I think many of the experts who recommend these procedures don't see the struggles that mothers go through down the road. I am not at all surprised that many mothers of premies give up. (In fact, I interviewed one expert on premature babies for an article on how these infants develop during their first year, and he told me that the number of premies who are breastfed for any length of time is so low that it is almost zero. He didn't seem to consider what factors or hospital routines might be causing these low rates.) I also have seen mothers with premature babies who "fought the system" and insisted on skin-to-skin, kangaroo care, refused bottles and pacifiers, and followed their baby's cues for feeding. Yes, sometimes these mothers and babies stayed in the hospital longer than those who gave bottles and followed the schedule. But they came home exclusively breastfeeding and usually continued with fewer glitches and problems.

Index

—— A ——

All purpose nipple ointment.......162
Antihistamine.............................183
Any periareolar incision.....106, 107
Artificial nipples.....6, 151, 165, 185
Asymmetric latch 21, 24, 26, 33, 35

—— B ——

Baby problems............................79
Birth control pill.113, 114, 115, 139
........................180, 181, 182
Birthing practices 62
Blessed thistle 131, 132
Blood loss..................................111
Breast augmentation...................107
Breast compression 8
Breast engorgement 76, 92, 163
Breastfeeding pillow 100
Breast reduction 106
Breast surgery 106, 147
Bromocriptine 111, 184

—— C ——

Cabergoline 111, 184
Cesarean section..........................69
Clamping down..........................51
Cleft lip 82, 85
Cleft palate 83, 151
Clicking.....................................56
Compression 129, 131
Cradle hold................................36
Cross cradle hold........................24

—— D ——

Decrease in milk production 181
Demerol......................................68
Diuretics...................................183
Domperidone....................137, 138
Doula 62
Drugs which decrease
        the milk supply 183

—— E ——

Early feeding cues......................23
Edema 2
Electronic fetal monitoring 63, 64
Endocrinologic syndromes.........110
Engorgement 76, 92
Epidural.............................2, 62, 66
Episiotomy 68

—— F ——

Fenugreek ..131, 132, 133, 134, 157
Finger feeding
        ....84, 152, 153, 155, 204
Flat nipples...........................73, 74
Football hold 34
Foremilk and hindmilk................18
Frequency of breastfeedings 8

—— H ——

Herbs do seem to help...............131
Human milk fortifier 171
Hypernatremic dehydration 105
Hypothyroidism 113

I

Improving the baby's suckle........37
Insufficient breast tissue.............116
Insufficient milk supply 103
Intravenous fluid 2, 64

K

Kangaroo mother care......9, 10, 165
........................166, 167, 171

L

Labor and birth intervention 90
Labor support...............................90
Lactation aid................................146
Lactation amenorrhea method....115
Large breasts 74
Latching on the premature baby ....
....173
Low blood sugars......................151

M

Maternal illness...........................184
Milk ejection reflex......................19
Mother with
        very large breasts 210, 211

N

Narcotic medication.....................68
Nipple and breast problems 73
Nipple confusion...........6, 7, 85, 93
Nipple pain.................................48
Nipple shields.......................77, 162
Nipple variations.................149, 150

P

Pacifiers.................................7, 169
Periareolar incision 107
Polycystic ovarian syndrome 112
Pregnancy.................................182
Premature babies....9, 12, 16, 70, 77

121, 139, 165, 166, 167, 168
169, 171, 172, 174, 175, 177
................................214, 215
Pseudoephedrine 184

R

Retained placental fragments
................................109, 147
Reverse pressure softening 2

S

Scheduling.................................187
Self-attach 3
Separation 70
Sheehan's syndrome 110
Side-lying...................................35
Skin-to-skin................................
....9, 10, 11, 12, 69, 154, 157
Sleep training 187
Supplementation 8, 91, 136

T

The mother's posture 37
Thrush 52, 53
Tight frenulum 50, 209
Tongue-tied 51

V

Vitamin K...................................11

W

Water, sugar water 8

Z

Zinc 198, 199, 201

Dr. Jack Newman graduated from the University of Toronto medical school in 1970, interning at Vancouver General Hospital. He did his training in pediatrics in Quebec City and at the Hospital for Sick Children in Toronto from 1977-1981. He became a Fellow of the Royal College of Physicians of Canada as well as Board Certified by the AAP in 1981. He has worked as a physician in Central America, New Zealand, and South Africa. He founded the first hospital based breastfeeding clinic in Canada in 1984. He has been a 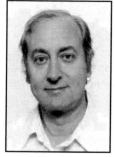 consultant for UNICEF for the Baby Friendly Hospital Initiative, evaluating the first Baby Friendly Hospitals in Gabon, the Ivory Coast, and Canada.

Dr. Newman was a staff pediatrician at the Hospital for Sick Children emergency department from 1983 to 1992 and was, for a period of time, the acting chief of emergency services. However, once the breastfeeding clinic started functioning, it took more and more of his time, and he eventually worked full time helping mothers and babies succeed with breastfeeding.

Dr. Newman has several publications on breastfeeding. In 2000 he published a help guide for professionals and mothers on breastfeeding called *Dr. Jack Newman's Guide to Breastfeeding* in Canada (revised edition, January 2003) and *The Ultimate Breastfeeding Book of Answers* in the US. In 2005, he and others brought out a DVD on breastfeeding called *Dr. Jack Newman's Visual Guide to Breastfeeding*.

Teresa Pitman is the mother of four children, all breastfed, and the grandmother of two grandchildren, also breastfed. She has been a La Leche League Leader for 28 years and is currently the Executive Director of La Leche League Canada. She is also a certified childbirth educator and doula. She writes for a number of parenting magazines and is the author or co-author of a dozen books on parenting topics, as well as a frequent speaker at parenting, birth, and breastfeeding conferences. Teresa lives in Guelph, Ontario, Canada.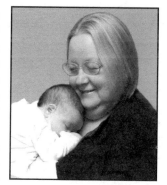

Ordering Information

Hale Publishing
1712 N. Forest St.
Amarillo, Texas 79106 USA

8:00 am to 5:00 pm CST

~

Call...806-376-9900
Sales...800-378-1317
FAX...806-376-9901
International (+1-806)-376-9900

~

Online Web Orders...
http://www.iBreastfeeding.com